SHINGLES

Thomas Carl Thomsen

Cross River Press * PO Box 473, Cross River, NY 10518 * 914-763-8050

Volcano Press * PO Box 270, Volcano, California 95689 * 209 296-3445

Library of Congress Cataloging in
Publications Data.

First Printing, May 1990
Second Printing, July 1990

Thomsen, Thomas Carl 1920 -
Shinglcs/by Thomas Carl Thomsen;
introduction by Benjamin L. Crue

p. cm
Includes bibliographical references

ISBN-945288-01-8: $17.95

1. Herpes zoster -- popular works.
2. Neuralgia -- popular works.
I. Title.
RC147.H6T46 1990
616.5 22--dc20   90-1305
                  CIP

Dedicated to my wife, Eleanor, and our
family for their invaluable support
in this very trying period of affliction

Also by the author:
Tales of Bequia, *Cross River Press,* 1988

CONTENTS

Introduction Benjamin L. Crue, Jr. M.D. ....Page 1

Chapter 1 My Bout With Shingles 5

Chapter 2 Some Commonly Held Myths 28

Chapter 3 It May Have Started With Job 32

Chapter 4 Viruses Are The Culprit 37

Chapter 5 How the Immune System Works 43

Chapter 6 You Are Not Alone 51

Chapter 7 What Is Shingles All About? 58

Chapter 8 How To Treat Shingles 68

Chapter 9 Can Shingles Be Prevented? 83

Chapter 10 PHN, The Worst of All Fates 89

Chapter 11 A Better Lifestyle is a Must 96

Chapter 12 Pain 107

Chapter 13 How to Treat PHN 121

Chapter 14 Can PHN Be Prevented? 132

Chapter 15 A Summing Up 135

Chapter 16 Post Script 139

Glossary 141

Bibliography 147

Introduction

Benjamin L. Crue, Jr., M.D., F.A.C.S.

Emeritus Clinical Professor, Neurological Surgery, University of Southern California School of Medicine, Los Angeles, California, and, presently, Medical Director of the Durango Pain Rehabilitation Center and the La Plata Community Hospital Regional Rehab Center, Durango, Colorado

As a neurosurgeon, with a lifelong interest in patients with chronic pain, I am now in my thirtieth consecutive year as a medical director of a pain clinic or pain center, either in California or Colorado. The medical specialty of treating patients with chronic pain syndromes, such as postherpetic neuralgia, is now referred to as "algology". As an algologist, I have been aware of many, many patients, with varied chronic pain sydromes over the years, who have sworn that their experiences were so horrible that when they got better they were going to write them up for posterity, either to satisfy an innate desire, or to let their family, or to let mankind in general, know what it's like to go through the suffering of a chronic pain syndrome. Unfortunately, very few patients ever do follow through and write such an epistle. Furthermore, of those who do, most of them, quite frankly, are so self-centered with the patient's own suffering (which horrible as it may be, is medically and psychologically the sine qua non of most chronic pain syndromes) where the patient's suffering becomes so much the center of his existence, and

1

his very being, that the literary product is often of very little interest to others. Having said this, it is with real feeling that I hasten to point out that the author of "Shingles," Thomas Carl Thomsen, is one of the very, very few exceptions. He has personally gone through the torment of not only acute shingles with its dermatological skin eruptions, but then the subsequent sequelae of post-herpetic neuralgia, and has, quite frankly, utilized the writing of this book as part of his own therapy of keeping busy, distracting himself from his own suffering, and has produced a volume that I personally believe has been very well researched, is very comprehensive, and is done in a clear literary style that makes reading it an interesting and informative experience.

The author spends very little time talking about his own particular case, other than to use it, quite properly, as an illustration. He has looked into many of the common myths that he's heard about shingles and postherpetic neuralgia, and has done good historical research, pointing out that the suffering (from Job on down) caused by shingles and postherpetic neuralgia is a matter of record and yet has not really been represented by much reporting in medical literature. He has gone to outstanding experts in the various medical fields for his facts about the nature of shingles, the incidence of the disease, ways of treating it, how a new vaccine may one day spell the end of shingles, the incidence and pathology of postherpetic neuralgia and ways of dealing with this nasty complication.

The author does a good job of pointing out that there are really two separate conditions; one is the acute viral infection that is usually referred to as shingles, with unilateral skin eruptions that can occur in any spinal nerve dermatome; or, in the cranial nerves, that may as in the authors case affect the first division of the trigeminal and lead to corneal scarring and blindness. The second is the condition of postherpetic neuralgia which does not occur in everyone, but most often occurs in the elderly or those with impaired immune systems.

Reflecting my experience with over 4,000 cases, postherpetic neuralgia is not correlated with the severity of the acute viral phase. It appears to be more apt to occur in the elderly, presumably because of impaired or destroyed afferent nerve pathways and resulting hypersensitivity, and because of a previous drop-out of sensory neurons due to age compounded by a new drop-out of neurons related to shingles itself. There is evidence that it may also be related to the chronic pain-prone personality traits of the individual, and to his available support systems, including family, religious beliefs, etc.

There is still a rather divergent point of view within the medical community as to whether postherpetic neuralgia represents the continued smoldering of a low grade infection; or, as I believe, the virus may well have long since become quiescent (although it may still be harbored in the tissues) and there is no need to postulate viral activity and ongoing nociceptive peripheral input sensory messages for the development of postherpetic neuralgia. This leads to the oft discussed conflict between the peripheral theory of chronic pain, versus the centralist concept that postherpetic neuralgia is one of the true chronic pain syndromes that requires only epileptiform firing in the central damaged deafferentiated neural sensory networks to explain both the neuralgia jabs of pain (that respond rather well to anti-convulsants) or the constant burning dysesthetic surface pain (that responds less well to antidepressants.) I personally believe that the treatment of postherpetic neuralgia is never surgical (and, indeed, surgical intervention should be considered "malpractice"); but, that postherpetic neuralgia can best be treated by support systems, including psychotherapy and chronic pain treating teams with experience such as are found in centralist-oriented pain treatment centers.

I am very grateful that the author of this book has presented both sides in an attempt to give the interested reader an impartial and fairminded view of the entire situation concerning postherpetic neuralgia. He is indeed to be congratulated. It is a pleasure to have read this manuscript, and I have been pleased to write an introduction.

Chapter 1. *My Bout With Shingles*

If you bought this book because you are into home repair, you made a mistake. This is a book about another type of shingles. The kind you would just as soon forget. If you had a choice.

I contracted shingles Labor Day weekend of 1986 and at this time I am still afflicted by its sequel, postherpetic neuralgia. It has been a dreadful experience. Only those who have gone through it can appreciate the degree of pain that is involved. I have a new understanding of the pain Job experienced, as described in the book of Job in the Old Testament, and a keener realization of the importance of patience and fortitude.

I am not alone in my suffering and perhaps that is some consolation. The number of people who experience the agony of shingles and neuralgia is substantially greater than most people realize. Medical researchers place that number at 1.2 million people, which is much higher than for many other more publicized diseases.

By comparison, there were 65,000 cases of AIDS in 1988, 250,000 of multiple sclerosis, and 985,000 new cases of cancer. Included in the 1.2 million new cases of shingles are about 108,000 who suffer from the nasty aftermath of shingles, postherpetic neuralgia, a condition that can last for years.

The incidence of shingles is even greater than the figures indicate. Each year the number of people who are affected increases by 1.2 million, so that in a twenty-year period about 24 million will have experienced the agony of a shingles attack—about 10 percent of the population. In the course of a 70-year lifetime, one out of five will have contracted it.

You would think, that with so many people affected, the medical community would have found a cure by now. A possible explanation is that shingles, while causing intense suffering, is seldom fatal. Other diseases like cancer and AIDS appear to have a much higher priority than shingles because of their terminal consequences. Also there are organizations actively promoting awareness of these diseases, while none exists for shingles.

I have learned a lot about the do's and don'ts of dealing with this disease and the purpose of this book is to pass on to fellow sufferers the experiences that I have had and the information that I have collected for their benefit. I hope others will also benefit. For example, wives, husbands, and children, whose support is essential to a smooth and rapid recovery. I hope it is not presumptuous to think that the medical community might also benefit. At least many of the doctors that I queried indicated that they would like to read the results of my efforts.

I doubt that I would have undertaken anything this complex if I had been able to find literature on the subject at the bookstore or public library. There were books on herpes in general and about herpes simplex, the cause of those familiar sores about the mouth, and sexually transmitted herpes genitalis, both of which have no connection with herpes zoster, the medical name for shingles. But I found nothing on shingles itself and so I began an investigation that has lasted for several years. In this period I collected medical journal reports published in the last twenty-five years dealing with shingles and postherpetic neuralgia and corresponded with researchers in government, university, pharmaceutical, and private laboratories to determine what the prospects are for better ways of dealing with the disease. I also conducted a survey of several hundred doctors to determine their experiences in treating the infection.

Shingles has several names. In the medical community it is called herpes zoster, or varicella zoster. The word herpes is onerous because of its association with other types of herpes such as herpes genitalis, which implies promiscuous behavior. For this reason a number of doctors prefer to call the disease varicella zoster, varicella being the virus that causes chickenpox and is also responsible for shingles.

My bout with shingles began when my wife and I and a cousin and his wife vacationed at Montauk the Labor Day weekend of 1986. We were having lunch in a lovely restaurant on the Sound side of Montauk when I began to feel a tickle in my right eyebrow. I thought that an insect had bitten me and that the sensation would pass. The next day we drove to Shelter Island, where we used to live, and the tickle continued and later in the day, when we were playing golf, the tickle became needle-like jabs, which were quite uncomfortable. When we returned to New York the following day, I made an appointment to see an opthamologist. I chose an opthamologist because the pain was around my eye and the internist whom I usually consulted was away. He took one look and gave me the bad news, that I had shingles and that I should consult with my internist who would return the following day. By now a rash had appeared on my forehead and close to my right eye. Because of the possibility that the virus might invade the eye itself and cause blindness, I was admitted to a hospital immediately and treated with acyclovir intravenously for a period of eight days.

By the time I entered the hospital six days had passed since the first indication of shingles, much too long a period for acyclovir to work at maximum effectiveness. Chances are that, if it had been administered promptly within seventy-two hours of outbreak, acyclovir in combination with prednisone might have prevented postherpetic neuralgia, the nasty sequel to shingles, when pain persists beyond a month.

Lesson one: don't treat the symptoms of shingles lightly. Get to a doctor at once. Hospitalization is not ordinarily indicated and is prescribed primarily when an eye is endangered, or when the infection spreads to other parts of the body and threatens to invade internal organs. Acyclovir is the drug of choice and is available orally, intravenously and topically.

Lesson two: be sure you have a competent doctor. In their responses to my survey, a number of doctors wrote that the best way of dealing with shingles is to let the infection run its normal course. If I had followed that advice, a number of complications could have occurred. The virus could have invaded the cornea of my eye and caused blindness, and the next target might have been the brain stem and then the brain itself. The resulting infection is called encephalitis, which results in brain damage or death.

My first stay at the hospital was a lonely experience because I was placed in quarantine. I was surprised at first, but then was told that shingles could induce chickenpox in a person who had not had chickenpox as a child, and to get chickenpox as an adult is a very nasty and serious experience. The quarantine was quite complete. In addition to the warning on my door, nurses had to wear special gloves and coveralls, which were discarded at the door and picked up later by an orderly. Visitors were asked if they had had chickenpox. They were admitted if they answered affirmatively. Otherwise they were turned away. The hospital floor was in a small panic when the nurse in charge learned that one of the nurses attending me had never had chickenpox. She was put off the floor and treated, I believe, with gamma globulin. She never returned while I was there.

I did not seriously mind being quarantined. I wasn't in any mood for visitors. I was a mess. My head was distorted, swollen on the right side and covered with sores. My right eye was closed. My son exclaimed when he saw me that I looked like elephant-man, an allusion to a disfigured wretch who was the subject of a Broadway play many years ago. When the surgeon, who had operated on me for cancer three years earlier, paid me a visit, he recoiled in shock and disbelief. Later I was told that mine was the worst case of shingles that the hospital had experienced. There was small comfort in knowing that.

The first two days were spent in and out of the

hospital's laboratories. A radiologist reported, "Erosion of the inferior aspect of one of the dorsal vertebrae bodies is present, probably due to a Schmorl's node." "No definite abnormality," was the result of a cat scan. The blood tests revealed nothing abnormal. A cardiogram indicated inverted T-waves but this corrected itself by the time a second cardiogram was made on discharge. Most of the tests were part of the hospital's routine and disclosed minor problems but nothing significant that had any bearing on my case of shingles.

The internist was more concerned than others when the sores spread to my chest. In his report, he wrote, "We are going to look for immunological problems and studies for gamma globulin disturbances have been ordered." I was glad that he was concerned because when shingles disseminates it can invade other parts of the body and cause considerable trouble.

His concern did not end when I was discharged from the hospital on this and then a subsequent occasion. Several weeks after the second hospitalization he told me that two of the hospital's six patients with AIDS had contracted the disease as a result of blood transfusions, which I had had at the time of my cancer operation. I submitted to the AIDS test and for ten days I waited anxiously and in suspense for the results. Fortunately, they were negative.

Some doctors describe shingles as a disease of the elderly. This is only partly true. The basic disorder is an impaired immune system. In addition to age, the immune system can also be affected by chemotherapy, radiation, the use of steroids, transplants, stress, diabetes and one's life-style.

The pain seemed manageable while I was in the hospital. I was discharged when the threat of dissemination into the eye and other organs of the body had been stopped and I was on the road to recovery. When the sores crusted, the pain really started. There were two types of pain. One was a burning sensation. The other was severe, lancinating, like electric shocks, the worst that I have ever experienced.

A variety of drugs was administered orally at home: prednisone, acyclovir, darvon, dilantin, and carbamazepine. It now seems like a mishmash of antiviral drugs, steroids, anti-convulsants, anti-depressants, and sedatives, all administered in a period of less than a month. The result, unfortunately, was that they did not work, and I was back in the hospital October 18 for "pain control and IV hydration."

The admitting doctor was a neurologist. In his admissions report, he wrote, "Tegretol will be discontinued. Allergic reaction. Start on diphenythydantoin." In his discharge report eleven days later, he wrote, "Given parenteral analgesia under supervision of a neurologist. Discharged under oral medication." The mission had been accomplished as far as the doctor and the hospital were concerned, which was to control the pain with injections and then to wean me off injections in favor of oral medication.

The second hospitalization was much more unpleasant than the first. I had to be given pain injections every four hours and the times when the nurses were off schedule, the pain became intense. The first hospitalization was a breeze by comparison. On the first occasion, I felt well enough after the sixth day to go home, but the doctor's views prevailed and I recall being rather annoyed at the time.

It is rare that shingles requires hospitalization once, let alone a second time. You might conclude that I have a low threshold for pain. But that is not the case. I can usually manage pain quite well and my recuperative powers are normally quite good. Until the bout with cancer, I had never been seriously ill, and I recovered quickly from that. As a matter of fact, I was on my way to the Caribbean with my wife within two weeks of discharge from the hospital.

By now shingles had taken on a new identity: postherpetic neuralgia. This is the name the medical community ascribes to shingles after the sores have crusted and healed and the pain persists beyond a month. It is difficult to explain this phenomenon. There are many theories but the facts are scant. One school of thought is that the pain is due to epileptic-like firing of pain impulses within damaged nerve circuits. Another is that the sensory nerve pathways have been damaged, affecting the pain modulating mechanisms. A third hypothesis is that a low level of viral replication continues long after the acute shingles is over. This view is plausible, although unproven, since complete immunity does not occur after a shingles attack and a susceptible person can have two and even three attacks later in life. Since the virus is always present in some state, it could be responsible for a continuation of the pain, which may last for many years after the initial attack.

In addition to causing considerable pain, postherpetic neuralgia, or PHN as it is sometimes referred to, produced other effects. My right eye was closed. The right side of my forehead and scalp, where the sores had appeared, was completely numb. I had no feeling whatever. I could not wrinkle my brow or raise or lower my eyebrow. And yet, strangely, the surface of my forehead and scalp were super-sensitive to touch. I could not sleep on my right side, shaving and brushing my teeth hurt, and the slightest breeze through my hair caused pain. Wearing a hat of any kind was out of the question.

How do you explain the seeming contradiction that my forehead was both numb and super-sensitive? Once again there are theories, but few hard facts. One possible explanation is that the sensory nerves, which lie at the surface, were inflamed causing pain, while below the surface the sensory pathways had been severely damaged and numbness was the result.

Alternating with the pain were periods of intense itching that affected the scalp, forehead, cheek and the right side of my nose. There is a theory that itching is basically a form of pain, and that different sensations such as itching, burning, and stabbing relate to the type of injury. I tried various medications to soothe the itching but none provided more than temporary relief.

There appears to be no standard explanation for what takes place in the postherpetic stage as the nerve system attempts to recover from the damage done by the virus. It can only be assumed that the large diameter nerve fibers, if not completely destroyed, are in the process of repair, that the pain modulating systems, which play an important role in controlling pain, are undergoing regeneration, and that the nerve endings on the surface of the body are being revived. These are only assumptions since there is no proof to substantiate them. It is probably because of this that current treatment is aimed at moderating the pain and not at restoring the normal functioning of the damaged nerve system. Why this is so is a matter that needs to be addressed by the medical profession.

I was discharged from the hospital October 29 and for the balance of the year I was treated with a combination of anti-depressants, anti-convulsants, and analgesics. It is interesting that, while not designed specifically for post-herpetic neuralgia, anti-convulsants and anti-depressants have proven partially effective for reasons no one seems to understand.

In this period I also tried nerve blocks and acupuncture. The theory behind nerve blocks is that after each injection of a local anaesthetic into the affected nerve center, the period of relief from pain would increase and ultimately the pain would disappear. I received ten nerve blocks over a period of about a month and the period of relief never extended beyond the initial three hours of numbness. I had a similar negative experience with acupuncture. After six unsuccessful tries, the acupuncturist explained that the procedure should have been started much earlier to be effective. This is questionable in the view of some neurologists.

In January of the following year I decided progress had been scant and that a new approach was in order. I consulted the head of the pain clinic at Montefiore-Albert Einstein in New York. The outcome was a change in medication to a combination of doxepin hydrochloride and trilisate. There was an unexpected fall-out benefit from the visit. The clinic head said there was no connection between alcohol and recovery, which contradicted the advice that I had been following. I had abstained from alcoholic beverages for a period of five months, and so naturally I was pleased by the new evaluation.

He also introduced me to Zostrix, a salve that had just come on the market. The salve is intended to ameliorate pain in the area applied. The primary ingredient is derived from hot peppers. One rationale is that it sets up a counter irritation to the one causing the pain. It worked reasonably well but I decided to discontinue it, because the smallest speck would cause considerable discomfort if it reached the eye. It would be less hazardous in cases where shingles invades the torso rather than the forehead and scalp. Even so the user is well advised to wash his hands thoroughly after application. Lioresal, an antispastic medication, was dropped at about this time. The stabbing pains had abated, leaving only the burning sensation to deal with.

By the end of January my wife and I were on our way to our winter home on the island of Bequia in the Caribbean. I must have looked dreadful. My right eye was closed and my face was badly scarred. I wore sun glasses in disguise and to protect my eyes against the sun. I did not feel great but I must have looked a lot worse. I learned later that a friend's wife, whom I had not met earlier, told her husband that she did not think that I was long for this world. I am glad that I did not hear her comment. Dealing with postherpetic neuralgia is a difficult struggle and what one needs is support at every step of the way.

I went about my business in as normal a way as was possible under the circumstances. I was doing research on a book and I was determined that my ailment was not going to interfere. I had to make concessions, however. The constant trade winds were an irritant to my eye and the ultraviolet rays of the sun caused the nerve endings on my forehead to flare up and cause pain. So I stayed out of the sun and dips into the lovely sea were short. I did find, however, that the seawater had a soothing effect on my eye. A doctor later explained that the composition of seawater is pretty much identical to the liquids that surround the eye.

I fully supported the view of the neurologist at Montefiore-Albert Einstein that alcohol would not impede recovery. An occasional rum punch helped to divert my attention from my ailment, and two or three were sheer bliss. Later this analgesic effect was confirmed when I read Dr. Mark Swerdlow's book, "Therapy of Pain," in which he points out that one drink is an irritant to a central pain mechanism but that several produce an analgesic effect. Three cheers!

I was fortunate in having considerable support from my wife, my son and his wife, my daughter and granddaughter who visited us at our retreat. I cannot overemphasize the importance of support. The danger of postherpetic neuralgia is that it tends to focus your whole attention on your dilemma and this then consumes your waking and sleeping hours. Attention and care from members of the family can help to offset the trauma and make one's life more tolerable and manageable.

When we returned home in April, I decided to consult an opthamologist about my eye, which was now open, but with a badly drooping lower lid. Ordinarily, the shingles virus confines its attack to sensory nerves. In my case it attacked the motor nerves around my eye as well and caused what is described as Bell's palsy.

We considered surgery as a means of bringing the lower eyelid back into position, but decided to wait a while longer to see if the lid would repair itself. The decision was a correct one. The eyelid regained much of its original function, although not entirely, and even to this day there are occasions when the lid will droop.

There was seldom a lack of activities involving the family to divert my attention from the ever continuing pain of postherpetic neuralgia. On returning home from Bequia, my wife and I learned that our granddaughter, Melanie, was planning to be married that June to a young man from Portugal. As the surrogate father, it was my responsibility to arrange for the wedding and reception. Fortunately, our daughter, Debbie, had attended to most arrangements while we were away and so there was little to do but enjoy the occasion. I gave the bride away reluctantly because we had been quite close and actually I thought of her more as a daughter than a granddaughter. While pain was still with me, it took a back seat to the more important moment at hand.

Family affairs never quite settled down into a nice,

uneventful routine. The following winter Debbie was infected with Lyme's disease and a month or so later Mike, my son, damaged his back at work, convalesced for several months, had a back operation, convalesced some more, and was out of work for almost a year.

The following year my wife fell and hurt her back and is in physical therapy at this particular moment. I had an arthroscopy on my left knee and this limited me for several months.

All of these family activities served one useful purpose and that was to distract my mind from neuralgia.

I was preoccupied for the balance of 1987 with a book that I was writing about Bequia. This in itself was good therapy. I continued on doxepin and trilisate, which seemed to moderate the pain. I say 'seemed' because progress was very slow, imperceptibly slow. The only way I could measure it was in the span of a year. By this time I had had shingles and PHN for more than a year, but there was no question that my health had improved.

In the fall I returned to New York University at Washington Square for a refresher course on fiction. This tied in with another book that I was working on, a mystery dealing with corporate intrigue. It had been over forty years since graduation and this prompted some introspection, which had many benefits, including being able to put PHN in a proper perspective.

I recalled some experiences I had with auto-suggestion during World War II and decided to give it a try. The discipline is relatively simple. You lie down, close your eyes, reduce the rate of breathing, and try to induce a state of complete relaxation. When the state is achieved, you suggest to yourself that your pain is diminishing and that it will soon disappear. I was surprised and pleased to learn that it worked more often than not, at least with regard to the burning pain on the surface of my forehead and around the eye. Unfortunately, it had no effect whatever on the stabbing, shock-like jolts of pain.

The possibility that one can control or at least moderate certain kinds of pain by auto-suggestion is supported by a group of algologists (pain specialists) who believe that some types of chronic pain are psychosomatic and should be treated psychologically. In their view this kind of pain is controlled by a central pain mechanism and trying to deal with it as peripheral pain is a waste of time. While this view is not a prevailing one, there is merit in the idea since the mind can have a significant influence on the degree of pain that is experienced. How else do you explain the placebo effect? In most scientific studies a group of participants is given a valueless medication, the purpose being to compare their responses with those given the medication being tested. There is inevitably a number of these participants who report benefit from the valueless medication. This is called the placebo effect. The explanation is that among this group are participants who believe fully in the benefits of the medication and have set their minds on improvement.

There are well over a thousand pain clinics across the country which offer their services to the sufferers of PHN. The acceptance of psychiatry as a means of dealing with pain is reflected in the staffing of many pain clinics, which usually include a psychiatrist, as well as a neurologist, and physical therapists on staff. Unfortunately, there is no accepted code of discipline for pain clinics, so their staffing, services, and medical concepts can differ widely, and it is not easy to select the one from which you would benefit most, or to weed out the medical hustlers, of which there are some.

When my wife and I returned to Bequia in January 1988, I felt better and apparently looked better. I had dropped from 185 pounds, my normal weight for many years, to 170 during the course of this illness. By now I had regained the loss and put on another 10 pounds. I felt somewhat overweight but did nothing specifically about it. In the course of time the excess weight melted off and today I am back to my normal weight.

The scarring on my forehead changed. The white splotches were tanned by the sun, but returned later when the tan vanished. The holes and crevices created by the sores were still there, although less visible.

I was busy. I completed the book on Bequia, which was published June 1, 1988. I also got started on the research for this book. Being busy is great therapy. My strong recommendation to anyone with shingles or PHN is to become involved in some activity that can consume a lot of time. If you don't have a hobby, get one.

When we returned to the States in April, 1988, I began spending time in the medical library of the New York Academy of Medicine on Fifth Avenue and 103rd Street. Getting to the library involved working my way across Spanish Harlem. My friends told me this was a risky operation, but I wasn't concerned, and I made the crossing many times without incident. As a matter of fact, I made so many visits to the academy that the hatcheck man called me doctor on arrival and when I left the doorman always referred to me as doctor and offered to hail a taxi. I got a Walter Mitty kind of kick out of being called doctor and did not try to correct them. The help I received from the librarians was particularly important at the beginning when I did not know my way around.

At about this time I switched from doxepin hydro-chloride to amitriptyline, another anti-depressant. The switch was made because I had been on doxepin for over a year and my neurologist felt that my body had built up a tolerance to the drug.

Why anti-depressants are effective is hard to say. The first to use an anti-depressant was an Australian doctor who felt that all of his shingles patients were depressed. He started giving them an anti-depressant and their ability to cope with the pain was much improved.

I tried a couple of therapies that I had read about in medical journals. I tried icepacks, which provided relief for the moment but had no lasting benefit. I had better luck with a vibrator, which I applied to my scalp and forehead several times a day. The theory behind the use of a vibrator is that it induces a counter-irritation, which helps to activate pain-modulating mechanisms in the nervous system.

I also discovered Mineral Ice, a new product on the market designed to relieve muscular pain. At the time of its introduction it was promoted as a means of easing various kinds of pain including shingles. Later this claim was dropped. I do not know why because it did help to soothe my forehead when the burning pain flared up. My wife was impressed with the results and gave it a new name, Miracle Whip. I still use the product and carry a small vial around with me at all times.

I realized a little late how important exercise is. As described later in this book, a group of Canadian doctors found that regular exercise improved the ability of their patients to cope with the pain of postherpetic neuralgia. It did not occur to me that exercise would have this benefit. I was limited because my forehead and scalp were super-sensitive to sun and wind. Golf was out of the question. I should have found alternate means of exercise but did not. The lack of exercise over a three-year period may also have had some bearing, I am told, on the fact that arthritis has crept into some of my joints.

It is now the spring of 1989 as I start to write this book. There has been improvement in my condition. My eye still smarts and my forehead and scalp are still tender and there are periods of intense itching. But for the first time in nearly three years I have been able to sleep on my right side. There is a slight pain when my forehead touches the pillow but it subsides as I settle into a sleep mode. The secret is to remain still and not shift about. So maybe I am in the homestretch and can look forward to a time sans PHN.

I continued on medication until late summer. I realized I should get off amitriptyline because I had become dependent on its sedating effect. The first two times I tried to quit were failures. Withdrawal resulted in jitteryness. The third time I was determined not to get back on it again and in time the uneasiness abated and finally disappeared.

My first step in collecting information for this book was to talk with the doctors who had treated me and they referred me to various medical journals, going back as far as 1965 when Dr. Hope-Simpson, a Britisher, published a comprehensive study on shingles. Reading the journals gave me sufficient background to be able to use Medicus and Medline, two data banks serving the medical community. At the outset, I thought there would be little information available, because I felt, as did so many others afflicted with shingles, that the disease was being overlooked by the medical community in favor of more urgent and critical diseases such as cancer and AIDS. I was partly wrong. I found more going on than I had expected but really not enough to satisfy me that real progress was being made.

I realized that for the book to be useful it would have to go beyond current practices and provide information about research work taking place and what the prospects were for uncovering new therapies and new approaches to preventing the disease. I wrote to researchers in government, university, pharmaceutical, and private medical institutions and received considerable information.

Among those who were most helpful were the School of Medicine of the University of Alabama, the American Academy of Dermatology, Burroughs Wellcome, Centers for Disease Control, University of Colorado, Columbia

University College of Physicians and Surgeons, Dana Farber Cancer Institute, DNAX Research Corporation, La Plata Community Hospital, Mayo Clinic, Merck Sharp & Dohm Research Laboratories, University of Minnesota Department of Laboratory Medicine, National Institutes of Health, Pfizer Central Research, Prevention Magazine, Sloan Kettering Memorial Hospital Pain Clinic, and Yale University School of Medicine.

The book will attempt to provide the reader with everything he should know about shingles and PHN and how to deal with them, to know what kind of help he should seek, to be able to monitor his own progress, and to learn what he can do on his own to promote recovery. Since I am not a doctor, I cannot advise medically, but I can provide sufficient information so that the reader can draw his own conclusions.

The chapters will cover myths about shingles and what the true facts are; history of the disease beginning with Job; identification of the people who are at risk; a description of the disease; an examination of viruses in general and varicella zoster in particular and how they work; the immune system and the role of DNA; the pathogenesis of shingles; the methods of treatment; prevention of shingles; a description of PHN; the role of nutrition; the meaning and control of pain; and the prevention of PHN.

There are many myths concerning shingles and one of the more disturbing ones is that shingles may be a forerunner of cancer, a commonly held view until recently. There is no connection other than that an impaired immunity system opens the door to viral attacks of all kinds.

In time shingles is likely to become a disease of the past. A vaccine has been developed to prevent chickenpox and is being tested among adults to prevent shingles. It is expected that the vaccine will be administered to children at the age of fifteen months in conjunction with vaccines for measles, mumps, and rubella. For that generation chickenpox and postherpetic neuralgia may cease to be a threat. Testing of the vaccine has been completed and Merck & Co. has filed an application with the FDA for a product license. The earliest date for its availability is sometime in 1990. In the case of adults, the usefulness of the vaccine to stimulate and reinforce immunity to the varicella zoster virus has not been fully proven and formal testing will probably not start until after it is licensed for use among children. If the tests are successful, the vaccine will probably be given at regular intervals at an early middle-age. A best case scenario is that it may be a matter of several years before it becomes available as a deterrent to shingles. For present sufferers, the vaccine may avert a second or third attack. A knockout blow to shingles will depend on the percentage of the adult population that consents to the vaccine. Adults who do not take the vaccine and get shingles will help perpetuate the cycle of reinfection by becoming agents for causing chickenpox among those who have not had chickenpox and are at risk.

Important as the development of the vaccine is, it does not diminish the need for a better medical understanding of shingles and postherpetic neuralgia and how to treat them effectively. In 1988 the National Institutes of

Health funded 31 projects at a cost of $3,478,271 dealing specifically with shingles and postherpetic neuralgia, a rather small sum considering the large number of people afflicted with the diseases. Only one of these projects dealt specifically with postherpetic neuralgia. Treatment will continue along present empirical lines, which has proven unsatisfactory, until the government is pressured to place a higher priority on shingles and PHN than presently exists.

A recent research report that will be described later in this book states that aspirin is more effective than most of the other remedies being used.

For the most part dealing with shingles and postherpetic neuralgia should be under the direction and control of a competent medical practitioner, such as an internist, dermatologist, or neurologist. Nevertheless, there are things that the patient can do on his own to accelerate progress and these will be discussed in detail. Here are a few highlights:

1. Get plenty of rest.

2. Exercise moderately. Take walks. Avoid strenuous exercises like running.

3. Cool compresses, calamine lotion, corn starch or baking soda may hasten the drying of the shingles sores. After the acute phase, a bland ointment of olive oil dressing may help soften and separate the crusts.

4. If the pain continues after the sores have vanished Zostrix and Mineral Ice may provide relief.

5. Avoid stressful situations and get the people around you to maintain a cool atmosphere and provide support.

6. Follow a balanced diet. Certain foods and beverages have an adverse effect on certain shingles sufferers. There are no precise guidelines. You can find out which ones cause your pain to flare up by experience. Included in this category are caffeine and chocolate. There are probably many more.

There are many foods that can strengthen your immune system. They are described in the chapter on nutrition.

7. If you have shingles on your forehead and around your eyes, protect yourself with a sun block and sun glasses and wear a loose fitting cap.

8. Don't hesitate to switch doctors if progress has come to a standstill.

9. Keep busy. Get a hobby if you don't have one.

10. Lastly, if you know someone who is showing signs of shingles, urge him to see a competent doctor at once. The severity of his attack can be moderated substantially if treated within seventy-two hours.

I hope this book proves helpful to you.

Chapter 2. *Some Commonly Held Myths*

In the process of collecting information for this book, it soon became apparent that there is a great deal of misinformation concerning shingles—what it is, how it is contracted, what connection it has with cancer and AIDS, how it should be treated, what complications can occur, and what the outlook is for developing a means of prevention. So, my first target is to try to set the record straight. Here are the more significant myths that I have encountered and what the real facts are.

Myth. The best way of treating shingles is to let it run its natural course.

Fact. This may be okay if you are young. But wrong if you are middle-aged or older. Arthur Rubinstein, the famous concert pianist, was told this, suffered greatly, and was obliged to cancel an important concert tour. Today, there are remedies. A combination of an antiviral drug and a steroid may shorten the period of infection, reduce the pain, and possibly limit the risk of getting postherpetic neuralgia, which can be even more painful than shingles.

Myth. Shingles is a nervous disorder.

Fact. The implication here is that shingles is an emotional disorder and probably should be treated by a psychiatrist. Shingles is a viral infection that invades nerve cells and causes inflammation and severe pain, and should be treated by a qualified internist, or dermatologist. If it develops into postherpetic neuralgia, it would be wise to consult a neurologist.

Myth. Shingles is a forerunner of AIDS.

Fact. The likelihood of this happening appears to be confined to homosexuals. In their case shingles may represent an early warning sign of impending AIDS.

Myth. If the shingles rash spreads about your body and forms a complete circle, you are likely to die.

Fact. This was once a commonly held opinion, but it has been disproven. Furthermore, the rash seldom covers both sides of the body. The myth may have had its origin in cases in which the infection had disseminated to other areas of the body. There can be serious complications in this event, but death is seldom one of them.

Myth. Shingles can lead to cancer.

Fact. This is another theory that was widely held in the medical profession at one time, but it has been discarded. The link between cancer and shingles is that both have a common cause, a damaged immune system. There is another possible connection. A nerve root damaged by cancer can open the door to an attack of shingles.

Myth. Shingles is the result of cancer.

Fact. One's immune system can be damaged by the use of chemotherapy and radiation in treating cancer and this could increase the risk of getting shingles. But cancer is not the cause of shingles.

Myth. People who have or have had shingles are more likely to get rheumatoid arthritis, diabetes, multiple sclerosis, and Parkinson's than those who have not had shingles.

Fact. Studies have shown that there is no proof of a link between shingles and these diseases.

Myth. Shingles is related to herpes simplex, an infection around the mouth and lips, and herpes genitalis, and implies loose behavior.

Fact. These infections are linked only by name. They are distinctly different. Some doctors prefer to refer to herpes zoster (the medical name for shingles) as varicella zoster, dropping the word 'herpes' and avoiding the confusion.

Myth. Shingles can last for years.

Fact. Shingles usually lasts less than a month. If pain persists for a longer time, shingles has developed into postherpetic neuralgia, which is treated very differently from shingles, and can last for years.

Myth. Shingles are infectious.

Fact. You cannot catch shingles from a person infected with shingles. But an adult or a child, who has not had chickenpox, can catch chickenpox as a result of exposure to shingles. It is not a likely possibility, however, since transmission requires skin contact. For an adult to get chickenpox is often a very serious matter and can be dangerous.

Myth. Shingles seldom leads to anything that seriously threatens health.

Fact. If not handled properly and quickly, shingles can lead to postherpetic neuralgia, encephalitis, pneumonitis and keratitis. It can cause death, but this is a remote possibility, except in cases where the pain becomes so severe and intractable that suicide becomes an alternative solution.

Myth. There is nothing that the family can do to help.

Fact. Support by the family is essential. In its

absence, a victim of the disease can become despairing and this can aggravate the disease and delay recovery.

Myth. The pain of postherpetic neuralgia is mental.

Fact. It depends on what one means by mental. Certainly, the mind plays a role in that a positive attitude, elimination of stress, and quiet meditation can help control the pain. But it is not a disease of the mind.

Myth. The medical profession is doing little to find a means of preventing the infection.

Fact. A vaccine developed by the Japanese is in use today in Europe and Japan, and is being tested in the United States and may be available in 1990. The vaccine is designed to prevent chickenpox. This is important because the varicella virus that causes chickenpox remains latent in the body and may erupt later as shingles. The use of the vaccine on adults as a deterrent to shingles is presently being researched.

An area of great promise involves the engineering of the DNA of infected cells to block the virus. Attention is also being directed at the role nutrition plays in strengthening the immune system.

Chapter 3. *It May Have Started With Job*

It is known that shingles has been around since ancient times. But there is not much in print about famous people who have been afflicted by the disease. With its connotation of promiscuity, it probably was not the kind of thing that our forefathers liked to talk or write about. A review of the diseases of famous people will turn up many examples of leprosy, epilepsy, tuberculosis, and even syphilis, but few of shingles. There are a few exceptions worth noting.

A case can be made that Job may have been the first person of record to be tormented by shingles. Victor Robinson, in his essay in the History of Medicine, writes that "Job was afflicted with a general eruption of sores, causing great itching and severe pain, discoloration of skin, tending to cause swelling of the eyelids and closure of the eyes." A pretty good description of trigeminal shingles affecting the opthalmic nerve.

Verse 19, Line 17, Job says, "I am repulsive to my wife, loathesome to the sons of my own mother." Verse 30, Line 16, Job says, "Days of affliction have taken hold of me. The night racks my bones and the pain that gnaws me takes no rest." Earlier it is stated in the Book of Job that Satan went forth from the presence of the Lord and afflicted Job with loathesome sores.

Some historians have taken the position that Job was afflicted with leprosy. That seems doubtful, for Job finally recovered from his ailment, which would not be likely in the case of leprosy. Besides Job lived to the age of 140, according to the Old Testament. Leprosy takes its toll in far less time than that.

One of the literary giants, Jonathan Swift, author of Gulliver's Travels and a prolific writer and satirist, was not reticent about his bout, or possibly bouts, with shingles. Harold Williams, in his Collection of the Correspondence of Jonathan Swift, wrote, "From the end of March 1711 until the middle of September Swift has many references in his journal to the severe attack of shingles from which he was suffering." A. L. Rowse, in his biography of Swift, writes, "Strain of overwork and anxiety was getting to him. In addition to his frequent attacks of giddiness, in April he was laid out by shingles, the details of which he goes into unsparing detail."

Rowse's comment is particularly interesting because he places the blame on overwork and anxiety. Many doctors today are inclined to gloss over them as primary causes and are more disposed to describe shingles as an infection of the aging. Swift was only 44 at the time he was afflicted and he lived on to the age of 78, when he became insane and died.

Swift may have had more than one bout. In May of the following year, 1712, he wrote to Archbishop King, "When I had the honor of your Grace's letter of March 27, I was lying ill of a cruel disorder, which still pursueth me, although not with as much violence, and I hope your Grace will pardon me if you find my letter to be that of one who writheth in pain."

Warriors certainly were not immune to the disease. Dr. Reuben Friedman describes an affliction affecting

Napoleon Bonaparte as dermatitis herpetiformis. That could translate as a herpes-like infection of the skin. Sir William Fergusson, leading surgeon in London, went to France to examine Napoleon III in 1856. He wrote that Napoleon was afflicted with a range of ailments including neuralgia.

This is not intended to be a historical treatise, so I will confine myself to one more example, Arthur Rubinstein, the great concert pianist. He was with friends celebrating the 80th birthday of his good friend, Darius Milhaud, in Geneva. Rubinstein writes about this experience, "I complained during dinner about a little spot on my right cheek which worried me. The next day, the whole right cheek had a rash. A doctor in the American Hospital declared that it was shingles. An abominable, indescribable pain ensued but there was nothing one could do about it. It was heartbreaking to ask Hurok to postpone eleven concerts in America. I was sitting in a daze for long hours not daring to move my head."

A rash developed on the other side of Rubinstein's face the eve of a gala party for the wife of Baron Alain de Rothschild. A doctor mistakenly diagnosed this as chickenpox. Shingles remained with him. He attended the opening of "Pippin," a musical in New York in which his son starred. Rubinstein wrote, "I was completely oblivious to my shingles. By now they did not interfere with my playing but continued their hold on me as before and after."

The doctor at the American Hospital in Geneva was completely wrong. By this time much was known about the disease and how to treat it. That was not true in the time of Napoleon Bonaparte. Chickenpox was confused with smallpox and nothing was known of the connection between chickenpox and shingles.

Medical progress really starts with Richard Bright who in 1831 recognized the implications of the way the shingles rash is distributed in a belt-like swath across the body. The rash had to have its origin in a nerve center that affected a specific area of the body, or a dermatome. The nerve center is called a ganglion and there are many distributed on both sides of the spine and they affect specific dermatomes. Some thirty years later E. Von Barensprung in an autopsy discovered hemorrhage and inflammation in sensory ganglia and nerves of the chest after a shingles eruption. A study by Henry Head and A. W. Campbell in 1900 included post-mortem examinations of 20 persons who had had zoster. It was a monumental study. It described the acute inflammation and hemorrhaging of infected ganglia and sensory nerves, and the nerve damage linking the nerves to the sensory nerve endings and centrally with the spinal cord and brain.

The association between chickenpox and shingles was noted a few years later in 1909 by J. Von Bokay and was confirmed by a number of observers, including K. Kundratitz in 1925. The concept that zoster represents reactivation of latent varicella virus was first proposed by J. Garland in 1943, refined by R. E. Hope-Simpson in 1965, and recently proved by molecular analysis of viruses recovered from infections. In 1952 T. H. Weller and M. B. Stoddard succeeded in growing the varicella virus in a tissue culture system and T. H. Weller in 1954 showed that the virus was the same whether it came from a case of varicella or a case of zoster.

Since then medical attention has been directed at finding remedies and ways of preventing the infection, or at least controlling it.

Since shingles has been around for a very long time, it may seem strange to the afflicted person that the remedies now available are not as sure-fire as he might like them to be. After all, there are positive cures for diseases like syphilis and tuberculosis, and smallpox has been effectively eliminated. There may be an answer in the fact that shingles, like cancer and AIDS, is caused by a virus and only in recent years has the medical community begun to get a handle on how to deal with viruses.

Chapter 4. *Viruses Are The Culprit*

For many years doctors have been aware of viruses, but they could not be seen or identified until the development of the electron microscope in the 1930s. With this new instrument, which focuses and then electronically amplifies beams of electrons instead of visible rays of light, scientists could peer into a world that until then they could only assume existed. What they found was astounding, a world so small and complex that it boggled the imagination. They had been able to identify bacteria with conventional microscopes. But now they discovered a microorganism so small that hundreds of thousands could fit within the space of a single bacterium. They learned that this new organism was very different from bacteria. It was not living. It did not move about, eliminate waste, or divide, none of the characteristics of life.

Viruses are similar to bacteria in that they are parasites. But they do not compete with bacteria for food. Instead they invade a normal cell and attempt to take over. Bacteria compete with normal cells for fluids and nutrients. Viruses, however, invade cells and remain there and take over control.

With the electron microscope, scientists were able to define the sizes, shapes, and structures of viruses and to place them in groups. There are over fifty related viruses in the herpes category. Some infect only oysters, others are confined to chickens, turkeys, frogs, mice, squirrels, monkeys, and rabbits. Within this family of viruses, there are six that infect humans. The best known is varicella zoster. Others include herpes simplex, herpes genitalis, Epstein-Barr virus, which causes mononucleosis, and cytomegalovirus, which causes mental impairment in infants. The varicella zoster virus was found to be large in relation to other viruses, highly complex in structure, and surrounded by a protective envelope.

There has been signficant progress in recent years in understanding viruses and the diseases they cause. New molecular technologies are leading to a better understanding of the molecular biology of viruses. We now have a picture of the varicella virus. According to Drs. Jeffrey M. Ostrove and Genevieve Inchauspe of the National Institute of Allergy and Infectious Disease, it is 150 to 200 nm in diameter with an envelope bearing glycoprotein spikes. The center of the virus contains a nucleic acid core surrounded by a protein covering, within which is the viral complex of chromosomes. The virus possesses a double stranded linear DNA of approximately 125,000 base pairs, which is sufficient to encode about 75 proteins.

The varicella virus, like other viruses, is wholly dependent on you, the host. Once inside a cell, its apparent inactivity is replaced by an enormous expenditure of energy. Unlike bacteria, which are able to live most anywhere in the body, viruses are able to operate in only one environment, and that is inside an invaded cell.

An event as important as the perfection of the electron microscope was the development of ways to produce cell-culture systems. This allowed researchers to grow cultures of live cells and to introduce viruses for examination and experimentation. They could now observe the way in which a virus invades a cell and takes over its management.

Nucleic acids within a virus are the agents that take over control. These agents can force the normal cell to ignore its own life-support functions and compel it to direct its energies at reproducing copies of the virus. Essentially what happens is this: the genetic code that regulates the functioning of the normal cell is replaced by the genetic code of the virus and from this moment on it is a slave to the virus and its energies are under the control of the virus.

The body contends with viral invasions in a number of ways that will be described later in this book. In the case of the varicella virus, it would appear that there is a delicate stand-off between the virus that is latent in the nerve ganglion and the antibodies of the immune system. As long as the immune system functions properly, attacks by the virus are quickly repulsed and there is no infection. But let the immune system falter, the virus is reactivated and moves in and attacks, and, ergo, shingles.

DNA, an abbreviation for deoxyribonucleic acid, is the repository of hereditary characteristics and the reproductive components of chromosomes and viruses. It contains deoxyribose, which is found in the nuclei of human, animal and vegetable cells and is loosely bound to protein. It is the instrument within the virus that directs the attack of the virus on healthy cells.

The DNA core of the zoster virus, which is icosahedral in form (twenty faces), is the control mechanism of the virus. The virus burrows into a normal cell, takes over the functioning of the cell and orders it to produce more virus-infected cells. The invaded cell bursts, releases new viruses to infiltrate other cells and replicate further.

The DNA of all cells, healthy or infected, is made up of two long and twisted strands. Each strand is composed of four genetic encoding chemicals called nucleotides (adenine, thymine, guanine and cystosine) and deoxyribose and phosphate. The sugar and phosphate molecules form the helix shaped strands, while the nitrogenous bases connect the strands (adenine connects with thymine and guanine with cystsine). The nitrogenous bases instruct the genes to direct the synthesis of thousands of enzymes and other proteins within the cell. The order and combination of these four chemicals along the DNA backbones carry all of the information of heredity.

Each human cell contains about six feet of DNA strands, coiled and packed into 46 tight bundles of chromosomes, and each DNA is made of six billion base pairs of adenine with thiamine and guanine with cystosine.

The genome of varicella virus (the genome is the total gene complement of a set of chromosomes) contains 70 genes distributed about equally between the two DNA strands. The genes are organized compactly with very little overlapping between protein-coded regions. The origin of replication is located within the major repeats.

With our knowledge of DNA, we can understand how a virus works and how genes can be engineered and recombined to block the replication of a virus. The possible application to shingles is mind-boggling. It is the basis for the successful development and use of antiviral drugs, which stop viral replication by adding an antiviral block at the end of a DNA chain which cannot be matched. We are only beginning to understand how to manipulate the DNA for beneficial purposes. Dr. Stephen E. Straus, head of the Virology Section of NIH's Laboratory of Clinical Investigation, wrote in response to a letter from the writer: "It is theoretically possible to alter the DNA of a dormant varicella infected cell so as to prevent virus replication. To do so would require the development of gene therapy technology, which is still in its infancy."

The functions of the body are well integrated and coordinated like a complex, sophisticated guaranteed-for-life piece of machinery. It is truly a marvel the way the pieces fit together and work. The body is sometimes described as an adaptive mechanism that makes frequent adjustments as conditions change. But sometimes some part of the system balks and begins to function "for its own good," a concept described by David Bakan in his book, "Disease, Pain and Sacrifice." The idea can be applied to viruses. They replicate usually when some part of the defense system goes awry and functions contrary to design and purpose and "for its own good." Similarly, the DNA of a normal cell can be blocked from fulfilling its purpose when a specific gene, a renegade gene, takes over and dictates the occurrence of a disease, an abnormality, a contrary course of development. Fortunately, the concept can also work for mankind's benefit. Anti-viral drugs work because they induce a new factor to be added to the DNA of a diseased cell that prevents replication.

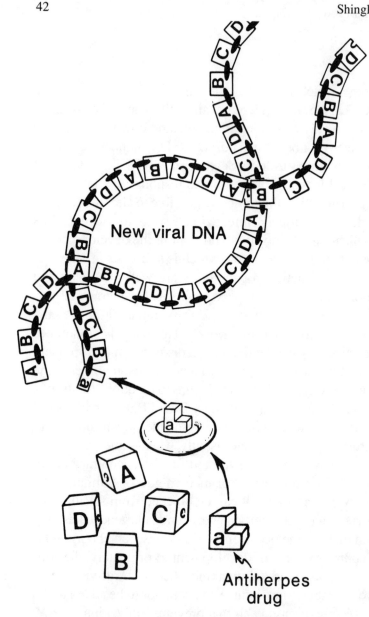

How many antiviral drugs work. As the double-stranded herpesvirus DNA is being formed by matching blocks, an antiviral block "a" is picked up by the doughnut-shaped DNA building enzyme and inserted at the end of the chain. Normal DNA building blocks won't match because of the irregular configuration of the antiherpes drug, and viral DNA cannot be completed.

Reprinted from "Effective Therapies for Herpes Disease," by Dr. H.H. Balfour, University of Minnesota Health Science Center, University of Minnesota Press, 1984.

Chapter 5. *How The Immune System Works*

One out of five people will get shingles at least once in a lifetime, while others will not. Why? The answer lies in the body's immune system, which works exceedingly well for most people but not for those whose systems have been impaired one way or another, by age, cancer, radiation, chemotherapy, transplants, diabetes, stress, to mention the major causes. There are ways to strengthen the immune system but for the moment let's look at the way it works.

The body's immune system is a complex of forces that has developed over a period of millions of years and reflects the influences of both heredity and environment. The effect of heredity is generally considered unalterable. As no two people look alike, genetic differences explain why no two people are exactly alike in their inherent ability to resist infection and fight disease.

The capacity and function of bone marrow, the lymph system, the thymus gland, and the trillions of cells that defend each person are unique to that person.

The body is under constant attack by viruses, bacteria and other parasites that fill the air and try to gain a foothold in the body by way of such entries as the nose, mouth, eyes, ears, and skin. Fortunately, they are almost always repulsed by a system of defenses: the toughness of the skin, the mucous of the nose and throat, tears and saliva.

If they succeed in penetrating these defenses, they enter the blood stream, multiply, and begin destroying vital body cells. Now the immune system goes to work.

Inside the body trillions of cells that are designed specifically to give battle are called to action. They are able to identify the invaders and they attempt to gobble them up. Some cells are constantly exploring the blood stream looking for foreign invaders. Other early warners direct the production of unique killer cells.

When the immune system is functioning properly, it is a difficult barrier for intruders to break through. Even in a setback, the components of the system are able to regroup and launch a counterattack. But sometimes the immune system fails to launch a counterattack quickly enough to be effective and an infection develops that will spread until sufficient antibodies can be created to knock out the disease.

The body's attack system includes macrophages, monocytes, neutrophils, T lymphocytes, and B lymphocytes, which work together as a well organized team. Macrophages originate in bone marrow and when they are released into the blood stream they are ready to attach themselves to virus-infected cells and devour them. T-lymphocytes develop in the thymus, a small gland in the neck, while B-lymphocytes are believed to originate in the lymph system at either end of the intestinal track. They are referred to as B-cells because they were first recognized in the intestinal lymph organ known as bursa in birds. Although they wait in readiness in the lymph nodes, a small number move back-and-forth between the lymph and blood streams searching for intruders. Plasma cells are transformed B-cells that produce special chemicals called antibodies that fight foreign invaders.

Neutrophils are among the first to arrive on the scene. There are about 126 billion neutrophils produced in the body daily. Produced in the bone marrow, they engulf the intruders and seek to digest them. But their life span is only a matter of days, so backup teams are called into action. A group of about 20 proteins are released into the blood stream, seek out the invader, cling to it, setting off a chain reaction that eventually kills the intruder. Macrophages, which are long-lived, now migrate through the body, locate the virus, engulf and then consume it, and send out a signal to T-cells to join in the fight. The T-cell is the captain of the resistance force. The macrophage secretes interleuken into the T-cell, which causes T-cells to replicate. The T-cells now release lymphokines, including gamma interferon, which stimulate the proliferation of phagocytes and macrophages. Simultaneously, other T-cells in the lymph nodes couple with B-cells and stimulate them to reproduce and to mature into plasma cells which now start to produce antibodies. Circulating in the blood stream, the antibodies seek out the virus and attach themselves to the virus and send out a signal to the macrophages to attack. The gamma interferon released by the T-cells serves a double purpose: it stimulates the macrophages to multiply and attack and also to stop or at least slow down the replication of the virus.

Now they attach themselves to a virus infected cell, punch holes in the cell membrane by shooting protein molecules into it which demolish the cell. The T-cells assure victory by sending a signal that forces the infected cell to destroy the DNA of the cell and the virus.

It is an intricate, well-organized and well-executed battle campaign. The immune system marshalls and employs its forces faster than the virus can replicate. As the effectiveness of the T-cells, B-cells, lymphokines, phagocytes, macrophages, plasma, and interferon reach a peak, it becomes too much for the virus to contend with and viral reproduction ceases and the viral infected cells collapse and the mopping up job is now left to the macrophages, while the other battlers return to lymph nodes, thymus and intestines where they originated. The regeneration of tissues and the healing process now start. In most cases of shingles healing is completed within a month of the start of the infection. If shingles develops into postherpetic neuralgia, it may take months and even years before healing is completed.

The immune system undergoes change as it develops experience with intruders. During the first encounter, detection works in a non-specific way. Thereafter, the immune system reacts to specific challenges, because it has retained experience from the first encounter. If the challenger turns up again, its presence will be detected instantly and specifically and the system's counterattack will be quicker and more effective. This feature helps to explain why in the case of most diseases once you have had it and recovered from it, future attacks will be moderate. In the case of shingles, most individuals do not experience a second attack, and if they do, it is usually mild.

Most diseases are the result of attacks by specific germs or viruses, but for the germs and viruses to be successful the body's immune system must be in a weakened condition. And it can be weakend by a number of events, such as age, chemotherapy, radiation, diabetes, transplants, steroids. When the body's immune system is weakened, it is prone to general as well as specific attack. The findings of Dr. L. E. Hinckle and a group of associates from Mt. Sinai Hospital indicate that the condition of being ill is a general characteristic of the total body and that the particular form that the illness takes is secondary. They concluded that a person with any one illness is more likely to get another disease, even in a remote body system, than a person who has had no illness. This can be translated to mean that a person with shingles should examine the general state of his health, because the conditions that brought on shingles might bring on other illnesses.

The role of the immune system is being recognized more broadly as a causative factor of sickness. It is particularly important in the case of shingles since exposure, the primary cause of disease generally, does not appear to be a major factor.

The effect of age on immunity is evident at all stages of life. At birth the only immunity a child has is what has been transferred by the mother, which is adequate usually until its own immune system develops. The system is at peak performance from childhood to early middle age, except for the occasions when we are exposed to microbes found in our environment, like cold viruses. But as we get older the effectiveness of the immune system wanes. For example, flu can be life-threatening to the elderly, while it is not particularly dangerous to young people. In laboratory tests it has been demonstrated that the responses of lymph cells by virus antigens (antigens stimulate the production of antibodies) decline with advancing age.

Another important factor is heredity. Genetic differences explain why no two people look alike and why immune responses differ from one individual to another. Dr. Richard Hamilton explains this phenomenon in his book, "The Herpes Book," as follows, "Because there is a core of inherited influences on resistance, there are individual differences in the various organs, glands, and other components of each person's immune system; therefore the capacity and function of bone marrow, the lymph system, the thymus gland, and the millions of cells that defend each person are unique to that person and are not subject to change."

There is much that is still unknown about the immune system's responses. Why is there such a long period of many years between having chickenpox and getting shingles? There is a theory that the zoster virus makes occasional assaults throughout one's lifetime, but the immune system fights back and develops more antibodies to forestall further attacks. This continues until later in life the antibodies wane and the next attack of the virus is successful and shingles results.

This theory suggests that shingles can break out at any time that the immune system falters and helps to explain why shingles is not totally confined to the aging and can attack younger people including children. In the case of young children, it is presumed that the immune system has not developed to the point of being able to control the disease.

Researchers are giving increasing attention to the role that the mind plays in the way the immune system functions. There is evidence that the way we think and feel can influence our ability to resist and fight infections. It is uncertain whether a positive attitude is ingrained in one's personality, or if it can be acquired and nurtured. It is probably both. I was able to function well most of the time except for the first month, probably because I am an optimist by nature and do not easily accept defeat. But I also learned that to an increasing extent I could control the burning pain by inducing a state of complete relaxation, blocking everything out of my mind, reducing the rate of breathing and suggesting to myself over and over again that the pain would soon subside. It worked more often than not, except in the case of stabbing pains, which required medication.

The immune system is also affected by malignant diseases such as cancer and leukemia, by immuno-suppressive drugs such as corticosteroids, and by radiation, chemotherapy and stress. As a consequence, the rate of shingles is high in patients with cancer and among patients who have been receiving immuno-suppressive drugs. For example, in one survey shingles developed in 35% of patients with Hodgkin's disease and in 8% of patients who underwent renal transplants. Patients with acquired immune deficiency are also likely to be at increased risk. The association between malignancy and the risk of zoster was interpreted for many years to mean that patients with zoster are more likely to have an underlying malignancy. This assumption has been disproved. The reverse, however, is true.

Chapter 6. *You Are Not Alone*

Probably everyone who has had shingles has asked himself, "Why me?" The pain is so excruciating and debilitating that there must be a reason why you have been picked to suffer. Are you being called on to do penance? For what? Are you a modern day Job whose faith and ability to withstand punishment are being tested? Many thoughts run through your mind. Some help your resolve. Others undermine your will to resist. All that you know is that when the experience is over you will know more about yourself, your strengths and your frailties, and your ability to manage yourself in exceptionally difficult circumstances.

Perhaps there is some comfort in knowing that you are not alone. Far from it, as a matter of fact. The medical community's estimates of the number of people afflicted range from 325,000 to 1,200,000 annually and that in the course of a seventy-year lifetime one out of every five persons will contract it. If you live to the age of 85, half of the people in your age-bracket are likely to have had shingles and four percent will have had it more than once.

A population-based study of herpes zoster and its effects was done by a group of doctors at the Mayo Clinic headed by Dr. M. W. Ragozzino in 1982. The study involved 590 residents of Rochester, Minnesota, who contracted varicella zoster in the 15-year period from 1945 to 1959. The study revealed that the incidence of shingles was 1.3 per 1000 person-years. Applied to a national population of 250,000,000 that would indicate that 325,000 people suffer from shingles in any year.

An earlier study by Dr. R. M. McGregor placed the incidence at a higher level of 4.8 per 1000, indicating that some 1,200,000 people are afflicted annually.

The study by Dr. Ragozzino's group also disclosed that:

The incidence rate was higher for women (23%) than for men (21%).

The incidence rates increased with age. They were lowest in the 14 years and under age and highest among individuals 75 years or more.

There was no evidence of seasonal trends. The incidence rates increased with time, rising by 41% for men and 28% for women from the 1945-1949 period to the 1955-1959 period.

In more than half of the cases (56.4%) the chest was affected. Next, in order of frequency, were the head (13.4%), the waist (12.7%), the neck (11.2%), and the pelvis (4.4%). In only 1.8% of the cases had zoster disseminated to other parts of the body.

The average age of patients with zoster of the head (56 years) was significantly greater than the rest of the cohort (46 years).

Complications affected 12% of the group. Postherpetic neuralgia was most frequent, occuring in over 9% of the patients. The duration of postherpetic neuralgia ranged from four weeks to greater than 10 years, with 22% having it for more than one year.

Of the 55 individuals with herpes opthalmicus, 20% had ocular involvement. Four were diagnosed with uveitis, three with keratitis, two with secondary glaucoma, one with iridocyclitis, and one with panopthalmitis. Six patients experienced motor deficiencies following herpes zoster, and five had Bell's palsy following facial nerve involvement.

Just over 5% experienced a subsequent episode of herpes zoster during the period of follow-up and two patients had two recurrences each.

Although people of all ages may be afflicted, there is a definite correlation between increasing age and the incidence of shingles. As we get older, our immune system undergoes change and becomes less effective in containing the virus.

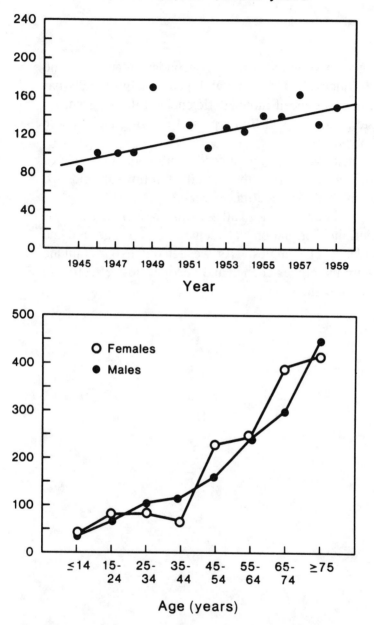

Incidence per 100,000 person-years of herpes zoster among residents of Rochester, Minnesota, 1945–1959, by individual year   (rates not age-adjusted).

Population-Based Study of Herpes Zoster and its Sequelae, M.M. Ragozzino, M.D., L.J. Melton, M.D., L.T. Kurland, M.D., C.P. Chu, M.S., and H.O. Perry, M.D., Medicine Vol. 61, No. 5, 1982.

OCCURENCE OF ZOSTER ACCORDING TO AGE

Age	Number of cases	Rate Per 1000 in each age group per annum
0-9	6	0.74
10-19	10	1.38
20-29	17	2.58
30-39	18	2.29
40-49	23	2.92
50-59	37	5.09
60-69	38	6.79
70-79	27	6.42
80-89	16	10.10

Varicella-Zoster Virus Infection, Charles Grose, M.D., and Roger Giller, M.D., University of Iowa, College of Medicine, CRC Critical Reviews in Oncology/Hematology, Vol. 8, Issue 1, 1988.

Incidence of Herpes Zoster Among Residents of Rochester, Minnesota, 1945–1959, by 5-Year Time Periods and Overall

	1945–1949		1950–1954		1955–1959		Total	
	N	Rate*	N	Rate	N	Rate	N	Rate
Male	61	107	73	113	110	151	244	126
Female	90	117	110	127	146	150	346	134
Both	151	112	183	120	256	150	590	131

* Incidence per 100,000 person-years, age-adjusted to the age distribution of the 1970 United States white population.

Complications of Herpes Zoster Observed Among 590 Residents of Rochester, Minnesota, 1945–1959

	Rochester		Burgoon (1)
	N	%	%
Post herpetic neuralgia	55	9.3	9.7
Motor deficit	6	1.0	
Herpes gangrenosa	3	0.5	1.0
Pneumonia	1	0.2	
Meningoencephalitis	1	0.2	0.5
Unilateral deafness	1	0.2	
Ocular complications	11	1.9	6.0
Uveitis	4	0.7	
Keratitis	3	0.5	
2° glaucoma	2	0.3	
Iridocyclitis	1	0.2	
Panophthalmitis	1	0.2	

Risk Factors Among the 590 Residents of Rochester, Minnesota, Diagnosed with Herpes Zoster 1945–1959

	Number	Percent
Cancer before diagnosis	36	6.1
Trauma	11	1.9
Radiotherapy	9	1.5
Chemotherapy	2	0.3
Systemic steroids	2	0.3
Surgery	1	0.2

Population-Based Study of Herpes Zoster and its Sequelae, M.M. Ragozzino, M.D., L.J. Melton, M.D., L.T. Kurland, M.D., C.P. Chu, M.S., and H.O. Perry, M.D., Medicine Vol. 61, No. 5, 1982.

LOCATION OF HERPES ZOSTER INFECTIONS AMONG RESIDENTS OF ROCHESTER, MINNESOTA, 1945-1959

	Number	Percent*
Head	73	13.4
Neck	61	11.2
Chest	307	56.4
Waist	69	12.7
Pelvis	24	4.4
Disseminated	10	1.8
Not known	46	—
	590	100.0

*Percent of known

Population-Based Study of Herpes Zoster and its Sequelae, M.M. Ragozzino, M.D., L.J. Melton, M.D., L.T. Kurland, M.D., C.P. Chu, M.S., and H.O. Perry, M.D., Medicine Vol. 61, No. 5, 1982.

Chapter 7. *What is Shingles All About*

A good place to start is with the meaning of the word 'zoster'. Zoster is derived from the Greek word for 'girdle', which describes the belt-like distribution of the rash across and around the body. The Swedish 'baltros' and English 'shingles', the latter derived from the Latin 'cingulus', have a similar meaning. In Europe shingles is often described as 'zona'.

The descriptions hardly do justice to the intense pain that is associated with shingles. They actually understate the distressing and debilitating effects that shingles can cause. Dr. Marcia Tonnesen, a dermatologist, describes shingles as one of the most difficult, distressing, and frustrating problems in modern medicine.

The pathogenesis of shingles starts with chickenpox, which affects most children and some adults. The varicella virus begins as an oral or respiratory infection. The virus is transmitted from the skin to nerve cells that are clustered together near the spine called dorsal root ganglia. There the virus remains dormant until such time that the immune system of the body undergoes change and breaks down.

Dr. R. Edgar Hope-Simpson, one of the pioneers in the field of epidemiological research, explains the phenomenon in the following way: "Soon after the initial attack of varicella, most of the sensory ganglia in the body begin harboring, for the rest of their lives, a harmless component of varicella pro-virus—fifty or more foci of incomplete virus, all of them liable, now and then, to revert to full infectiousness. Now and again one latent virus component will revert. Usually nothing perceptible happens. The minute dose of infectious virus which results is immediately neutralized by circulating antibody before it can multiply enough to cause perceptible damage. Even such a tiny encounter of antibody with virus may stimulate the immune mechanisms to produce yet more antibody. If, however, antibody has declined below the critical value necessary to blanket the explosion, at the next reactivation infectious virus will be able to multiply, perhaps at the expense of the nuclei of the satellite cells in the ganglion, setting up the most intense inflammation. The infectious virus is then transported antidromically down the sensory nerve, causing in its passage a fierce neuritis and neuralgia, and is released around the sensory nerve endings into the skin to produce the characteristic clusters of zoster vesicles."

If the immune system is inadequate to contain or repel the virus, the infection can spread to other sensory and sometimes motor nerve roots, causing further inflammation and degeneration. The infection can spread along the posterior nerve roots to the membranous envelope of the spinal cord and cause inflammation of the spinal cord.

According to Dr. Michael Oxman, the ganglion shows intense infiltration of lymph cells, necrosis (destruction) of nerve cells and fibers, proliferation of lymph-lining cells, hemorrhage and inflammation of the ganglion sheath. He states that some degree of nerve degeneration and infiltration of lymph cells is generally present in adjacent ganglia on the same side of the spinal cord.

Four to five days before the rash the patient may feel anything from numbness and tingling, itching, or burning to severe pain. When the virus reaches the skin, it erupts in clusters of blisters, which later crust and disappear. At this point the lesions no longer contain viable virus. In most cases the lesions usually resolve in two to three weeks. But the pain continues and the affected area is so sensitive that it is difficult to wear clothing or to find a comfortable position in which to sleep.

The discomfort can be continuous or intermittent. The pain is usually described as continuous aching or burning, often with severe lancinating electric-like jolts. It is sometimes mistaken for appendicitis, gallbladder attack, myocardial infarction, glaucoma, or pleurisy. Once the rash appears, the problem of diagnosis disappears. If the pain cannot be ameliorated, the patient may exhibit changes in mood and behavior, with diminished appetite, sleep disruption, and social isolation.

There are several explanations for the severe pain that is produced by shingles. A generally accepted one is that pain is caused by activation of pain sensors by direct viral attack and by inflammatory changes in nerve endings on the surface of the skin and in the dorsal root ganglia, nerve roots and spinal cord. It is also believed that the loss of sensory nerve fibers could contribute to the sensation of pain. Another theory is that the loss of large nerve fibers could allow for increased transmission of painful nerve stimuli through the dorsal horn of the spinal cord.

In addition to pain, the area of the body affected may become numb, a condition that may last for years, and alternating with the pain an intense itching that can be as troublesome as the pain.

The sores are not broadly distributed as in the case of chickenpox and are usually confined to a single nerve-area of the body called a dermatome. The affected area is usually along the course of one of the nerves beneath the skin. Most of the time only the sensory nerves are involved. Occasionally motor nerves are affected, as in the case of shingles around the eye, when the functioning of an eyelid can be temporarily impaired. When the rash is particularly severe, there may be superficial gangrene with delayed healing and subsequent scarring consisting of white areas where the nerve endings have been severely damaged.

Most sufferers from zoster recover without residual symptoms, except for scarring of the skin. An attack does not confer immunity and it is possible for a second and third attack to occur primarily among the elderly. Recurrence affects about 4% of patients and about half in the same location.

Although the virus usually affects a specific area, or dermatome, it is not uncommon for a few vesicles to appear in areas remote from the affected dermatome. The disseminated lesions usually appear within a week of onset, and if few in number they are of small consequence. More extensive dissemination usually occurs among patients who have immunologic defects due to an underlying malignancy or to therapies involving drugs that suppress the immune system.

Motor paralysis occurs in less than 5% of patients

with zoster and is the result of the spread of the virus from the sensory ganglion to nerves that control motor action. The rate of occurrence in patients whose cranial nerves are affected is significantly greater, usually in the range of 10 to 20%. Paralysis usually starts within two weeks of the appearance of the rash and almost always affects muscles that are contiguous to the dermatome involved. Functional, if not total recovery occurs in most cases, although considerable time may be involved.

The incidence and severity of shingles is greatly increased among patients who have or have had certain types of malignancy, such as Hodgkin's disease and leukemia and have used immuno-suppressive drugs such as corticosteroids, or have been involved with radiation treatment. Almost 50% of patients with Hodgkin's disease develop herpes zoster, with the highest incidence occurring in patients with advanced disease and those receiving chemotherapy or radiation. The severity of the disease is substantially increased and dissemination to other parts of the body usually occurs. One out of 10 patients with disseminated zoster develops widespread visceral infections, particularly of the lungs, liver and brain. At this point the disease can be life-threatening.

The occurrence and severity of shingles is also markedly increased in renal, cardiac, and bone marrow transplant recipients. In the absence of the use of antiviral drugs, old lesions may fail to heal and there can be periods of new lesion formation. Patients with AIDS are particularly vulnerable to repeated assaults by the virus.

There is another possible link between varicella

zoster and AIDS, which has been under investigation. A review by a group of 10 doctors, headed by Dr. A. E. Friedman-Kein, involving 300 patients with AIDS, revealed that 8% had prior zoster, a rate that is sevenfold greater than historic controls of the same age. All in the review group were homosexual men between the ages of 24 and 52 with no prior history of blood transfusions or drug use. The medical team arrived at the conclusion that the development of shingles among high-risk individuals may represent an early clinical sign of impending AIDS.

The precipitating causes of shingles are numerous. In addition to those already mentioned, Sir John Walton wrote in Brain Diseases of the Nervous System that "zoster may be precipitated by intoxication with various poisons, and may occur in the course of infections such as pneumonia and tuberculosis or toxic states such as uremia. It may complicate any lesion of the dorsal roots and can therefore follow fracture-dislocations of the spine, secondary carcinoma of the vertebral column, meningococcal and other forms of meningitis, subarachnoid hemorrhage, prolapsed disc, and spinal tumor." Other medical researchers have suggested ingestion of lead and arsenic, exposure to ultraviolet light, syphilis, and trauma as possible causes.

An important factor affecting vulnerability to shingles is a person's life-style. Most everyone has learned the role that adequate rest, a proper diet, and the absence of stress have on well-being. We are well aware of the effects of smoking, excessive drinking, and drugs on health. Lung cancer, heart disease, liver damage, and emphysema are examples of a life-style that has gone awry.

Stress is probably more damaging to one's immune system than any other feature of an individual's life-style. It directly impinges on the immune system because of the effect that hormonal surges brought about by stress have on antibody formation, lymphocyte function, and macrophage activity, all important activities within the body in resisting disease.

Dr. Hamilton explains the effect of stress this way: "The implications of stress-induced immune system depression for people who have herpes are clear: since the control of recurrences depends on immune status, any factor that lowers it can cause more difficulty." In addition to lowering immunity, the nervous agitation that accompanies stress may stimulate viruses to leave nerve tissue where they have been lying dormant, according to Dr. Hamilton. Controlling stress, therefore, is fundamentally important.

Shingles can have many complications, one of the nastiest being postherpetic neuralgia, which occurs in about 9% of patients in general and rises to 50% in the case of patients 60 years of age. Postherpetic neuralgia is the condition that exists after the rash has disappeared and the pain persists beyond a month of the start of the infection. The pain may resolve itself in a matter of months but sometimes can take years before it fully abates.

Shingles around the eye has a relatively high complication rate. The eye is involved in about half of the patients with opthalmic zoster. When the opthalmic division is involved vesicles appear on the forehead but the cornea may be attacked when the vesicles also appear on the part of the nose supplied by the nasociliary branch. Complications include retraction of the eyelid, keratitis, scleritis, glaucoma, palsy and optic neuritis.

Another complication is inflammation of cerebral arteries which may occur weeks to months after an episode of opthalmic zoster and may manifest itself as an isolated cerebral infarction, multiple infarctions, or a stroke in progress. Recurrences after the first few weeks are rare and the disease appears to be self-limiting. The mortality rate in reported cases is about 15%.

A most serious complication is herpes encephalitis, which is infection of the brain. This occurs when the virus moves from the trigeminal ganglia along nerve pathways leading to the brain. Its earliest symptoms include fever, headaches, changes in personality, speech problems, perceptual difficulties, muscle aches, and general weakness. As the infection spreads, the symptoms worsen, leading to seizures and eventually coma. Spontaneous recovery is rare. Fatality occurs among 70% and those who survive are left with permanent brain damage.

Another complication is myelitis which is inflammation of the spinal cord.

An extended bout with shingles and postherpetic neuralgia can result in severe depression because of the unrelenting pain. In some cases suicide is a viable alternative to continuation of a condition that offers little if any prospect of correction. Family support is absolutely essential to preclude this conclusion.

A doctor who is supposed to be an authority on

shingles writes, "No magic potion or lotion exists for shingles. For the most part, it is one of those live-with-it propositions, a waiting-out of the natural course of events as blisters dry. The limit of treatment usually consists of trying to ease the pain." What an understatement! If you have shingles and this is your doctor's advice, you should consider getting a second opinion and quickly before it is too late. As we have seen thus far, it is a very serious ailment with the possibility of serious complications if it is not attended to properly.

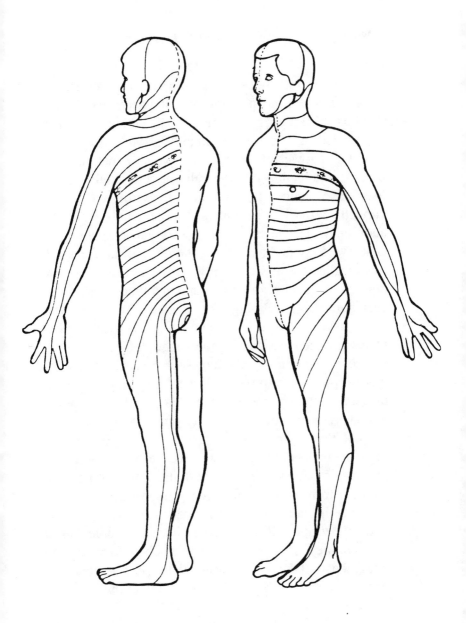

Dermatomes of the left side of the body, with shingles rash in one dermatome.

Chapter 8. *How To Treat Shingles*

It is generally believed that shingles has been around for a very long time, perhaps thousands of years. How is that possible? Dr. Hope-Simpson had a theory which he expounded at a lecture on June 19, 1964. It goes as follows: "How can we explain the paradox that the host-parasite interaction that we call varicella could not by itself have secured the survival of the virus, and yet the varicella virus is still with us? There must be some additional mechanism of virus survival, and surely in zoster we have just such an adaptation. During the attack of varicella, the virus is not only shed to start an immediate new cycle, but also goes to ground in a state of latency in each human host. Biologically, the latent state is useless to virus survival unless, sooner or later, reactivation takes place, and the virus once again reaches the general environment of the host. The attack of zoster is surely the missing piece of the puzzle. The neolithic human communities, cut off from frequent intercourse with one another, would produce in twenty to thirty years a new generation susceptible to attack by the varicella virus. One of the older members of the group would develop zoster, and so provide infectious virus to start the little outbreak of varicella from which the new generation would receive, in its turn, the latent parasites. Indeed, in just this way varicella virus still secures survival in remote island communities. Zoster must, therefore, be regarded as an integral part of the host-parasite relationship, a secondary or tertiary state of the varicella virus infection."

This chain of events may be coming to an end. When the varicella vaccine is introduced, it should put an end to the original chickenpox infection and the nail in its coffin will be hammered in finally if the vaccine works on adults to prevent zoster.

Now we come to the $64 question: "How do we treat shingles?" Although there are many things that a patient can do on his own to accelerate recovery, the burden of employing the proper therapy falls on the shoulders of the doctor and his advice should be sought at every step of the way.

This does not mean that a good patient is necessarily a passive patient. It is important that you know as much as possible about this disease, so that you can discuss it intelligently with your doctor and your family.

Let's begin with a review of current therapies and defer for the moment what you, the reader, can do.

First, the goals of treatment can be defined as follows: one, to provide relief from the pain; two, to halt and finally end the infection; and, three, to forestall, if possible, the development of complications such as postherpetic neuralgia.

In the December, 1986, issue of Annals of Neurology, Dr. Russell Portenoy listed some of the early medications that were employed: epinephrine, pituitary extract, sodium iodide, diphtheric antitoxin, snake venom, smallpox vaccine, procaine, dehydroergotamine and tetraethylammonium chloride. Despite claims of success, Dr. Portenoy states that these treatments have not been substantiated and are not favored.

No benefit has been demonstrated for other early treatments such as applying X-ray treatment to the involved ganglia and short-wave diathermy. The use of electric current (TENS) to stimulate surviving nerve fibers has had some appeal, but, according to Dr. Portenoy, has never become popular due to difficulties in applying the therapy over a region of damaged skin. Autohemotherapy, which is the injection of a patient's own blood into his gluteal muscles, has been used occasionally since the 1920s without a theoretical basis for the procedure. Case reports have been made of other substances, such as griseofulvin, amitidine, and dihydroemetine, without scientific substantiation.

Most important is the success being encountered with the use of antiviral drugs. An early antiviral agent, idoxuridine, was evaluated in two controlled tests and was shown to be effective in reducing healing time and pain when mixed (5%) with dimethyl sulfoxide in an ointment. The results of the test were reported in the British Medical Journal in 1970.

This led to the development of other antiviral drugs such as leukocyte interferon, which interfered with viral RNA and augmented the immune system's response to the virus. Human interferon appears to be effective in reducing the incidence of postherpetic neuralgia, according to Dr. Michael Oxman.

Three properties place interferon at the forefront of antiviral drugs, according to a report by the National Institute of Allergies and Infectious Diseases: one, extremely high antiviral activity; two, broad spectrum of applications; and three, low toxicity. The manufacture of leukocyte interferon, however, is very complicated and expensive and consequently has had only limited use.

The most popular and effective antiviral agent developed to date is acyclovir, which can be administered orally, topically and intravenously. In the writer's case it was used intravenously because of the need for substantial doses to prevent the virus from reaching the cornea of his right eye and possibly causing blindness. This meant hospitalization. In most cases the drug can be administered orally on an out-patient basis.

Acyclovir has been particularly effective in treating patients whose immune system has been compromised by chemotherapy, radiation, and high doses of corticosteroids. Oral acyclovir is currently being used for these patients. Dr. Myron J. Levine of the University of Colorado Health Science Center reports that application of acyclovir as an ointment favorably influenced the course of varicella zoster in immuno-compromised patients, but he adds that it needs further testing.

Dr. Portenoy reports that the prompt administration of acyclovir intravenously shortens the duration of the shingles rash and ameliorates the pain. In cases when the use of the drug was discontinued, pain worsened. He suggests that oral acyclovir may provide a means of treating acute attacks in most patients.

Acyclovir has no significant side effects when taken orally but can cause serious toxic effects when given intravenously. Central nervous system toxic effects include jitteryness, lethargy, tremors and disorientation, mostly in patients with abnormal renal function. Renal toxity is caused by crystallization of acyclovir within the collecting tubules but this is reversible and can be prevented by vigorous hydration, according to Dr. Mark H. Sawyer of the National Institutes of Health.

Patients with opthalmic zoster are at increased risk for ocular complications. Several studies have shown that acyclovir lessens ocular complications and reduces the possibility of relapses of ocular inflammation.

The development of acyclovir is an example of the progress that has been made in learning how to engineer the functioning of cells. It works in the following way. The herpes-infected cell produces a chemical called thymidine kinase, which, in turn activates acyclovir and makes it attractive to the enzyme building the viral DNA chain. The enzyme then adds the acyclovir block at the end of the viral DNA chain, where it sticks like glue, preventing the chain from being completed and halting the formation of new viral particles.

Another antiviral agent is adenine arabinoside (marketed under the name Vidarbine), which, according to Dr. John D. Loeser, has been shown to hasten the healing in immuno-compromised patients, decrease the risk of disseminated zoster, and decrease pain. It has no apparent effect, however, on the incidence of postherpetic neuralgia. The drug has also been found to be quite effective against herpes keratis, which can develop when zoster invades the eye. In studies conducted separately by Dr. Peter Laibson of the Wills Eye Hospital in Philadelphia and Dr. Deborah Pavan-Langston at the Massachusetts Eye and Ear Infirmary in Boston, Vidarbine was demonstrated to be at least as effective as idoxuridine, with few side effects. In the case of encephalitis, which is the result of the virus invading pathways to the brain, it has been shown that if Vidarbine is administered early enough it can prevent death and radically reduce the incidence of brain damage in survivors. The study was conducted by a team of 20 investigators headed by Dr. Charles A. Alford and Dr. Richard J. Whitley of the University of Alabama.

In another study cytosine arabinoside failed to demonstrate any benefit and a controlled comparison of normal serium globulin and zoster immune globulin disclosed no apparent value in either.

Acyclovir, Vidarbine, and interferon all favorably influence the duration of new lesion formation and virus shedding, healing of lesions, and rates of dissemination to skin and viscera, according to Dr. Mark H. Sawyer of the National Institutes of Health. Advantages of acyclovir are its ease of application and lack of side effects. All three drugs reduce pain but only interferon and Vidarbine clearly reduce the duration of chronic pain associated with zoster. "Pain reduction remains an area where antiviral treatment is still not satisfactory," states Dr. Sawyer.

"Instances of severe central nervous system complications of zoster provoke debates about the relative merits of antiviral drugs compared with corticosteroid therapy," Dr. Sawyer continues. "Arguments favoring the former cite evidence of viral replication in the pathogenesis of these conditions, particularly in immunosuppressed patients. That neurological complications often develop after the skin lesions have begun to resolve suggests that immunopathologic processes are at play that may be inhibited by corticosteroids. In the absence of more data, we favor the use of antiviral drugs in normal and immuno-suppressed patients, when such complications occur during the acute phase of zoster infection."

A relatively new antiviral therapy involves the use of fluoro-5 iodoarbinosylcytosine (FIAC). A study in 1986 by a group of doctors headed by Brian Lylan-Jones demonstrated that FIAC is an effective antiviral agent that is therapeutically superior to Vidarbine when the drug is administered to immuno-suppressed individuals.

A new antiviral agent, now under study and not yet licensed in the United States, is phosphonoformic acid, which is designed to act against herpes viruses.

Another approach is to develop drugs that can induce the body to increase its own production of interferon. At this time no drugs of this category have been licensed for use.

Research studies have indicated the possibility that viruses can develop a resistance to antiviral drugs. The mechanism by which the zoster virus can become resistant is by mutation of the viral thymidine kinase, which is the enzyme that induces the viral DNA to add acyclovir to its chain.

Another and different approach to treating shingles is with corticosteroids, which have the ability to alter the immune response. Dr. Russell Portenoy reports in Annals of Neurology that several case reports suggest that treatment with adrenocorticotropic hormone or a steroid could benefit patients with acute varicella zoster. He states that a double-blind placebo controlled study of oral triamcinolone in 34 patients with acute zoster revealed analgesic efficacy without effect on lesion healing time. Of patients over 60 years of age, only 30% of those receiving the steroid had pain beyond two months, compared with 73% of the control group. Treatment with steroids, Dr. Portenoy concludes, appears to accelerate resolution of pain.

Steroids have also been administered by injection under the skin. Enthusiastic reports of large numbers of patients claim 80 to 100% success in treating acute zoster. But these are anecdotal reports and need to be confirmed.

Prednisone is one of the steroids that has been used successfully to provide relief. Its disadvantage is that it is also an immune suppressive agent and would serve to further reduce immunity among patients whose immunity has already been compromised as a result of chemotherapy, radiation and certain forms of cancer.

Dr. Richard L. Whitley, Professor of Pediatrics and Microbiology at the University of Alabama, reports, "In our trials of herpes zoster we are evaluating the effect of corticosteroids with and without acyclovir. This study (December 1988) is 50% completed and will require another two years before termination."

Other drugs that have been used to treat shingles are: carbamazepine, an anti-convulsant that is used to reduce paroxymal stabbing pain. Possible risks include depression, liver damage with jaundice, and interference with bone marrow production.

Amitriptyline, an anti-depressant that also acts as a sedative and provides pain relief. It can, however, cause confusion, disorientation and hallucinations. It is used when shingles has developed into postherpetic neuralgia.

Doxepin, an anti-depressant, has the same properties as amitriptyline and is used for the same purposes.

Amantadine hydrochloride, a dopamine drug, has been used to reduce pain.

Capsaicin (Zostrix), a plant derivative that alters neuropeptide concentrations in certain nerves, is effective in reducing pain. It is applied as a salve.

Dr. Benjamin Crue, director of the Durango Pain Rehabilitation Center, Colorado, believes that doctors generally have been too conservative in their use of morphine in treating pain from shingles. "Not only is there sound neuropharmacologic evidence that narcotics are effective with a central blocking mechanism," he writes, "but also the accompanying sedation and euphoria can be helpful adjuncts in the treatment of severe acute clinical pain."

A completely different approach involves the use of anaesthetics. The injection of carbocaine and other anaesthetics along the neural pathways to the affected sites has been employed for a number of years as a means of reducing and finally eliminating pain. The theory is that the period of relief following each injection will increase and that in time the pain will be completely eliminated. Dr. Russell Portenoy reported in Annals of Neurology that in an uncontrolled group of patients the effects were good with pain relief occurring within two weeks of onset with either a paraspinal block for neuralgia below the head or with a stellate ganglion block for cranial zoster. One to four blocks usually provided relief. The success rate dropped to 40% in neuralgia treated two weeks after onset. Time, obviously, is crucial. The writer had 10 injections of carbocaine in the stellate nerve in the neck which had no beneficial effect whatever. The program apparently was started too late, well after the beginning of postherpetic neuralgia.

Acupuncture has been tried but the results have been inconclusive. The writer underwent acupuncture treatment, but it failed, perhaps because it was applied too late.

There have been many favorable reports about the efficacy of vitamins, particularly vitamin C, vitamin E and vitamin B. Dr. J. N. Dixon of New York wrote in Skin and Allergy News that he had great success treating patients with 10 grams of vitamin C daily. Dr. Frederick Klenner of North Carolina treated eight shingles patients with injections of 2 and 3 grams of vitamin C every 12 hours and one gram orally every 2 hours. All but one of the patients experienced substantial relief within 72 hours. Dr. John G. McConahey, a dermatologist in New Castle, Pennsylvania, routinely gives his shingles patients vitamins C and B complex along with corticosteroids. He reports, "Seventy-two percent of the pain is gone after the sores have disappeared." He believes that vitamins C and B complex help the nerve cells regenerate and rebuild. "The substance that surrounds the nerve fibers is derived from these very same substances."

Dr. Richard Meehan and Dr. Samuel Ayres of the

University of Southern California School of Medicine treated a group of 13 patients, 11 of whom had suffered moderate to severe pain for over 6 months, 7 for over a year, one for 13 years, and one for 19 years. Vitamin E was given orally and a cream was applied directly to the skin. The vitamins helped 9 who experienced almost total relief, while the remaining 4 showed some improvement.

According to Irwin Stone, author of "The Healing Factor: Vitamin C Against Disease," vitamin C has been shown to stop shingles pain, dry out the blisters, and clear the lesions within 3 days of being administered through injection.

Dr. Juan N. Dixon of New York treated herpes zoster patients with oral vitamin C and got excellent results. In each case the lesions dried up within 2 to 5 days. Vitamin C works, according to Irwin Stone, because ascorbic acid enhances the body's production of interferon.

In his search for relief, the writer also tried vitamin B12 injections. Again he blanked out after a dozen injections. Too late he was told that the efficacy of vitamin B12 is wiped out when alcoholic beverages are consumed the same day, even moderately.

All of the reports of the usefulness of vitamin therapy are anecdotal and have not been supported by any scientific studies.

In summary, a number of drugs and procedures have been examined by researchers with mixed results, some quite positive as in the case of antiviral drugs but inconclusive in the case of other treatments.

While it is imperative that you consult a qualified

doctor as soon as possible when the first symptoms of shingles appear, there are some things that you can do on your own to improve your ability to cope.

According to Dr. Michael Oxman, the application of cool compresses, calamine lotion, corn starch or baking soda may hasten the drying of the shingles sores. Occlusive ointments should be avoided, he says, and creams containing corticosteroids should not be used. After the acute phase, a bland ointment of olive oil dressings may help to soften and separate the crusts.

Most important is following a life-style that places a premium on rest and relaxation, avoidance of unnecessary stress, a proper diet, and the development of a strong positive attitude towards your affliction.

Dr. Norman Greer, an English doctor, writes this: "Patients with a positive attitude are much more successful in coping with cancer and other diseases. The mind can help. It can also hinder."

I have experimented a little with auto-suggestion, which boils down to repetition of a positive statement, such as "the pain is beginning to subside and will go away," in an environment of complete relaxation, where the mind is a blank and breathing is reduced and controlled. It may sound a little far out but auto-suggestion has been around as a therapy for a long time and in my case has provided relief from low intensity burning pain. It has not had any effect on stabbing, lancinating pain. I cannot explain why. Its successful use depends on your willingness to believe in its effectiveness.

There's an exercise that illustrates how auto-suggestion works that was used by Emile Coué early in this century. It is a fun exercise but it is educational as well. Draw a large circle on a sheet of 8-1/2 by 11 paper. Tie a string of about 11 inches in length to a small weight about the size of a half dollar. Hold the string so that the weight is directly over the center of the circle. Concentrate your attention on the circle and let your eyes follow the outline of the circle continuously. Almost immediately the pendulum will begin to swing in an arc following the outline of the circle. What happens is that when your eyes follow the outline of the circle, a suggestion is conveyed to your brain, which it automatically implements. You must be completely relaxed and you must not try to exert influence over the pendulum. The power of suggestion is as simple as that.

Paul Emile Levy offers the following advice in seeking to implement the power of auto-suggestion: "Let us represent ourselves to ourselves, let us picture ourselves as we would like to be—vigorous, robust, overflowing with health. The greater the sharpness of outline of this idea, the more salient it is, and the more it assumes the form of an image, the better the prospects of its realization. What is well conceived will be easily realized."

The suggestion that we make to ourselves about shingles should be general at the outset. For example: "Day by day, in all respects, I am getting better and better." Then we should pass on to specifics, dwelling mentally on the improvement we would like to effect. "The pain in my forehead is getting less and less and soon it will disappear."

Giraud Bonnet describes a procedure in detail. "Isolate yourself in a room where no one will come to disturb you. Settle yourself comfortably in an armchair, or lie down on a sofa or bed. Close your eyes. Relax your body to the utmost, for this physical inertia favors mental passivity and renders the mind more accessible to suggestion. When your nervous energy is no longer dissipated in making movements or in other work, it will be concentrated in the brain, and you will be better able to devote it to the idea you wish to realize. At the outset endeavor to stop thinking altogether. Try to think of nothing at all for a time. Then direct your thoughts towards the idea which is worrying you and counteract it by its converse." He used stage fright as his example. Concern over shingles would do as well. "Repeat the process several times. Have a number of sittings every day—in bed at night just before you go to sleep, during the night if you happen to be awake, in the morning immediately after waking. If you carry out this plan with assurance and conviction, success is certain."

I have also had success with a vibrator applied to the area that is numb and where surface pain continues. The vibrator was used in a late stage of postherpetic neuralgia. Applied over a period of two months, it restored some feeling to the numb area and decreased surface pain. A medical journal report suggests the use of a cooling chloride spray. The writer opted against this therapy because of the proximity of the eye to the affected area, which could have been damaged by the spray.

Another suggestion (and for this you don't need a

couch): take some comfortable walks and become deeply interested in anything that will distract your attention from your ailment. Avoid stressful situations as best you can.

Chapter 9. *Can Shingles Be Prevented?*

This chapter should be of interest to readers with shingles for two reasons: one, taking comfort in the knowledge that your children and grandchildren may escape this nasty ordeal, and two, warding off the possibility of a second or third attack later in life.

There is research going on in laboratories across the country, seeking ways of preventing shingles. The increase in research activity is due to a number of factors. The country's aroused interest in finding answers to cancer and AIDS has accelerated the development of cellular research and this has had a fall-out benefit for shingles research. Knowledge of viruses and how they work has greatly increased in recent years and this had led to new paths of investigation, new concepts and new drugs.

An important breakthrough occurred in 1974 when Takahashi and his associates in Japan developed a live, attenuated varicella vaccine (Oka strain). The vaccine has been under study in normal adults and immuno-suppressed patients, as well as children, in Japan, Western Europe, and the United States, and has been licensed for use in several European countries and Japan. In response to an inquiry from the writer, Dr. Stephen E. Straus, head of the Medical Virology Section of the Laboratory of Clinical Investigation of the National Institutes of Health, wrote, "Clinical trials are currently being planned to vaccinate middle-aged and elderly individuals with a live attenuated varicella vaccine in an effort to enhance their immune responses to the virus and prevent zoster. It will be several years before the merits of this approach are defined." The letter was written in December, 1988.

The primary objective of the vaccine is to prevent chickenpox in children. There appears to be little doubt as to its effectiveness in this regard. If inoculation is widespread and if the resulting immunity is permanent, or if it can be boosted at later intervals, shingles may become a disease of the past within a generation.

There is some concern in the medical community that the effect of the vaccine may be to defer chickenpox to a later time in life. This would be counter-productive because chickenpox at the adult stage is far more serious and difficult to deal with than in childhood.

Dr. Robert W. Finberg of the Dana Farber Institute states in a letter to the writer, "Studies with the Oka vaccine strain indicate there is no increased incidence of zoster in recipients." This was confirmed by Dr. Anne Gershon, Director of the Division of Pediatric Disease at Columbia University, who has been responsible for coordinating vaccine testing. She writes, "The incidence of zoster does not seem to increase as a result of vaccination."

Dr. Henry Balfour is concerned by the possibility that a live vaccine has the potential to promote the growth of cancer. He speculates that a vaccine made up of only a part of the virus will evade the "major concern in the development of herpes virus vaccines—cancer from the vaccine itself."

Dr. Straus wrote in the Annals of Internal Medicine in 1988, "In normal children and adults the Oka vaccine has elicited superior immune responses and has fewer side effects than in immunosuppressed persons. The protective efficacy is good, lasts for several years, and the few vaccinees who develop varicella after community exposure have mild illnesses. In anticipation of universal vaccination, the Oka vaccine has been proven to be immunogenic when given with vaccines for measles, mumps, and rubella to children at 15 months of age."

Apparently, it may be necessary to re-inoculate at regular intervals to assure continued immunity, at least among adults.

The Oka vaccine is also effective in preventing chickenpox among adults who did not have the infection in their childhood. Dr. Straus advocates vaccination within three days of exposure.

Dr. Gershon responds to a question from the writer, "It is known that if someone who has had varicella is given a dose of vaccine, a boost in immunity to the virus may occur. Whether this could prevent zoster, however, can only be determined by a placebo controlled study involving large numbers of patients." Such studies are now underway. Dr. Gershon comments, "I am hopeful that the vaccine will be licensed for the prevention of varicella in about 1990."

Dr. Gershon states that the vaccine will be given to children at the age of fifteen months in conjunction with vaccines for measles, mumps, and rubella. In the case of adults, it will probably be recommended that the vaccine be taken at an early middle age and that it be repeated at intervals, perhaps five years, to boost immunity. The vaccine is not likely to become available as a deterrent to shingles for several years. Formal testing by Merck has not been started and probably won't be until after the company has been licensed to market the vaccine for use in preventing chickenpox.

Another approach to prevention is the development of a vaccine through genetic engineering and recombinant DNA techniques. This is still in the research stage. The advantage of a genetically engineered vaccine is that it eliminates the danger of creating the disease the vaccine is supposed to prevent.

The gene-splicing recombinant DNA method involves the following steps, according to Dr. Balfour:

1. The key herpes gene is dissected from the DNA chain.

2. The herpes gene is spliced into a circular piece of DNA called plasma.

3. The hybrid plasma is inserted into bacteria.

4. A bacterial colony producing herpes antigens is selected.

5. These bacteria multiply.

6. The herpes antigens are separated from the bacteria and purified as vaccine.

Some day it may be possible to alter the DNA of a dormant infected cell so as to prevent viral reactivation. This would require the development of gene therapy which is still in its infancy. Dr. Straus believes "it will be some decades before such an approach could be considered practical, ethical and safe."

Dr. Robert L. Coffman of the DNAX Research

Institute of Molecular and Cellular Biology responds to the question, "Can the immune system of an adult in his middle years be enhanced so as to limit his exposure to herpes zoster?" with the observation that the possibility of manipulating immune responses to infectious agents to maximize the protective immune response is the subject of intense research at the moment. "It is too soon yet to give a clear answer to the question. The mechanisms of normal regulation of immune responses are just beginning to be understood." The letter was dated in January, 1989. Dr. Robert Finberg of the Dana Farber Institute believes that the immune response could probably be enhanced but at this time (late 1988) only non-specific enhancers are available.

One of the new therapies developed in the laboratories involves lymphokines, which are proteins that monitor and regulate the immune system. There are many varieties. In the interferon group there are three—alpha, beta and gamma. Alpha itself has many varieties. Interleukens are similarly prolific. They perform many functions, including the reproduction of white and red cells in bone marrow. They are used in various combinations to boost the immune system against specific diseases. According to immunologist Dr. Leroy Hood of the California Institute of Technology, the lymphokines discovered so far are "the tip of the iceberg. In the truest sense, immunology is just in its youth."

Interferon is one of the more promising members of the family of lymphokines. Dr. Balfour describes the way they function as follows: "Herpes viruses cause production of natural interferon immediately after they infect cells. Interferon turns off synthesis of proteins during the early stages of viral replication. It also stimulates lymphocytes, which are vital in the defense against foreign organisms. Finally, interferon seems to prevent the newly formed virus from escaping and invading other cells."

Gamma globulin has been tested as a means of preventing or moderating shingles but has not proved effective. It has been used successfully, however, in preventing chickenpox among persons who have not had chickenpox and consequently run the risk of catching chickenpox as a result of being exposed to shingles.

Chapter 10. *PHN, The Worst of All Fates*

A common and dreaded complication of shingles is postherpetic neuralgia, which is an extension of pain after the sores have healed. Since shingles usually lasts less than one month, continuation of pain beyond this time is defined as postherpetic neuralgia. According to Dr. Straus, postherpetic neuralgia resolves within two months in 50% of patients and within one year for 80%. It can last as long as 20 years for the remaining 20%.

A population study made by a group of doctors headed by Dr. M. W. Ragozzino showed that in Rochester, Minnesota, where 590 residents had shingles over a 15-year period from 1945 to 1959:

1. Nine percent of the group developed postherpetic neuralgia.

2. Duration of the pain ranged from 4 weeks to more than 10 years, with 45% having neuralgia for less than 8 weeks, while 22% had it for more than a year.

3. The average age was 67 years.

The pain associated with postherpetic neuralgia is unrelenting. It is usually accompanied by a feeling of numbness in the affected area, inspite of which the surface of the skin is super-sensitive to touch, and a slight breeze in the case of neuralgia of the face and head can cause severe pain. Paradoxically, there is no feeling of pain, only numbness, when pressure is applied.

Itching is another symptom. According to Dr. Patrick D. Wall, itching is a form of pain. He explains in his paper, "Mechanisms of Acute and Chronic Pain," that the "brain extracts differences between closely related injuries and sets off differing sensations such as itching, burning, or stabbing and differing behavior such as scratching, rubbing or holding still." All three sensations and types of behavior are associated with PHN.

Consequences of the unrelenting pain of PHN are depression, anorexia, lassitude, constipation, diminished libido, and loss of sleep.

The incidence and severity of pain are related directly to age. A study by Drs. J. M. Demorgas and R. R. Kierland revealed that 50% at age 60 and nearly 75% at age 70 developed postherpetic neuralgia within a month or more following the rash. The rate of occurrence is greater for those with zoster of the face and head.

Pain in a patient whose immune system has been compromised as a result of chemotherapy, radiation, transplants, diabetes and steroid drugs is likely to be more severe and prolonged, according to Dr. Straus, and can lead to scarring and dissemination of the rash to other parts of the body. Dissemination can be defined as more than 20 lesions outside the primary affected area. It is rare in the normal patient, but common in the person with a suppressed immune system and may be accompanied by internal and neurological infection, substantially increasing the risk of morbidity and death.

Pain is usually restricted to the area where the rash occurred, even in cases where a few sores appeared outside the main affected area. It is severe, can cause morbidity, bring about changes in personality, and occasionally prompts suicide as a viable alternative. Unremitting postherpetic neuralgia has been described as one of the most difficult pain problems with which the physician has to deal.

There are many theories about what is occurring in the nervous system when postherpetic neuralgia evolves from shingles. One is that the nerve pathways have been severely damaged, affecting pain modulating mechanisms. Another is that the inflammation caused by the viral attack has not completely healed. Another is that the virus is not dead and continues to reside in the affected ganglion and is in constant competition with the immune system, causing continued inflammation and pain.

This was explored in a study by Drs. Abbas Vafai, Mary Welles, and Donald H. Gelden of the University of Colorado. To determine whether postherpetic neuralgia might relate to reactivation of the zoster virus, blood mononuclear cells of patients with PHN were tested for the presence of the virus DNA and proteins associated with the virus. The DNA was detected in the mononuclear cells of one patient and the virus-specific proteins were found in the mononuclear cells of two acute varicella patients, one acute zoster patient, and six elderly patients with PHN. In the case of the three elderly zoster patients without PHN, the virus-specific proteins were not detected. The study concluded that the findings strongly suggest that persistence, reactivation and expression of varicella zoster may result in PHN.

A postmortem conducted by Dr. C. P. N. Watson and a group of associates at the University of Toronto of a deceased patient who had suffered with PHN for five years disclosed that the appropriate dorsal horn had atrophied and that a loss of large diameter myelinated fibers at the dorsal root had occurred, whereas the dorsal root ganglia appeared normal, and there was no deficiency in serotomin, dopamine-beta-hydroxylase or substance P in the dorsal horn.

A school of thought is that the sensory nerves are permanently damaged as the virus travels from the ganglia to the skin during the acute shingles attack.

Dr. Russell Portenoy writes that from the limited knowledge of the abnormal changes associated with postherpetic neuralgia it seems likely that chronic changes follow the acute inflammation associated with shingles. He writes, "The presence of ghost cells and chronic inflammatory changes have been confirmed by pathological examination of dorsal root ganglia from patients with postherpetic neuralgia."

"The pathophysiology of postherpetic neuralgia may involve both peripheral and central mechanisms," he writes. "The observation of a preferential loss of large nerve fibers in a patient with PHN has led to the hypothesis that impairment of segmental pain modullating systems may play a role." Diminished large fiber function may allow increased transmission of pain information through the dorsal horn of the spinal cord, according to Dr. Portenoy. Another theory described by Dr. Portenoy is that PHN is a form of pain resulting from the loss of sensory nerve fibers due to the changes in central pathways induced by peripheral nerve and nerve root injury.

The development of PHN may relate to still other

factors. In a letter to the writer, Dr. Benjamin Crue of the Durango Pain Clinic writes, "Patients without a good support system at home and with a high degree of anxiety and who are overly concerned with their health (I hate to use the word hypochondria) are all apt to develop post-herpetic neuralgia, and these may be more important in the causation of a prolonged painful post shingles pain syndrome than anything else." In a subsequent letter he added, "These are trigger mechanisms that stimulate the damaged central cells into uncontrolled epileptiform firing, causing the sensation of pain."

David Balkan expresses a similar thought in his book, "Disease, Pain and Sacrifice." He points out there is accumulating evidence that the duration of illness among persons is associated with psychological indicants, that the more favorable the indicants with respect to the mental health of the individual, the shorter the duration of the illness. Put another way, he states that there is evidence that the psychological condition of patients is a good prognosticator of the effectiveness of medical treatment.

Location of the infection also has an important bearing on the severity and the length of infection. Dr. Crue writes, "There does not appear to be any question that patients with shingles in the first division of the trigeminal nerve in the forehead and around the eye are much more apt to have severe postherpetic neuralgia than patients who have it on the chest, abdomen, or extremities."

Dr. Balfour suggests the hypothesis that a low level of viral replication continues long after the acute shingles attack subsides. "Quite possibly," he writes, "varicella zoster viruses are continually raining down the nerve pathways, causing constant inflammation and pain and damage to the nerve cells.... . Eventually our immune system rids us of all new viruses and the painful damage resolves."

Dr. Allen Aksamit of the Mayo Clinic writes, "There is a great deal of speculation about the pathogenesis of postherpetic neuralgia, ranging from scarring and inflammatory changes unrelated to the virus itself to persistent expression of viral genes after the active zoster eruption."

Postherpetic Neuralgia by Site, Corrected for Age.

Area	Zoster	Neuralgia	
		Expected	Actual
Cranial	45	8.0	8
Cervical	50	7.7	11
Thoracic	163	22.3	19
Lumbar	39	5.2	4
Sacral	16	2.8	1
Total	313	46.0	43

HOPE-SIMPSON. J. Roy.Coll.Gen.Pract. 25:571-575;1975

Duration of Postherpetic Neuralgia by Age Groups

Age Yr.	No. Patients	No Pain		Pain							
				Less than 1 Mo.		1-6 Mo.		6-12 Mo.		More than 1 Yr.	
		No.	%	No.	%	No.	%	No.	%	No.	%
Less than 20	24	20	83	3	13					1	4
20-29	53	34	64	18	34					1	2
30-39	69	25	36	32	47	5	7			7	10
40-49	135	43	32	47	35	30	22	5	4	10	7
50-59	204	42	20	63	31	57	28	6	3	36	18
60-69	270	41	15	54	20	65	24	11	4	99	37
70 or more	160	14	9	28	18	32	20	10	6	76	47

DE MORAGAS. Archives Dermatology. 75;193-196;1957.

Chapter 11. *A Better Lifestyle is a Must*

We have dealt thus far with what is going on in research laboratories that may have an impact on preventing varicella zoster. There is much that we can do as individuals to strengthen our immune system and thereby ward off shingles attacks. Our life-style is of paramount importance and this includes the kind of food we eat, the amount of rest that we get, and the way we live.

What is required is an expanded awareness of the way we treat our bodies. We are very vulnerable to disease and if we are not in top shape we stand a good chance of succumbing to diseases like shingles.

Victor H. Lindlahr wrote several decades ago that we are what we eat. The kind of food we consume supplies our body's 100 trillion cells with the fuel they need to operate effectively and the 100 billion plus army of macrophages, lymphoblasts, plasma cells, and T and B cells that are essential to our well-being.

In his Golan Memorial Lecture delivered February 13, 1985 at the North Shore University Hospital, Cornell University Medical College, New York, Dr. Ranjit K. Chandra, pediatrician and immunologist at the Memorial University Hospital of Newfoundland, presented the following view: "Nutritional deficiencies, excesses, and imbalances influence specific components of the immune system. The severity of immunological impairment depends upon the extent and nature of undernutrition, the presence of infection, and the age of onset of nutritional deprivation."

Dr. Richard Hamilton in his book on herpes observes, "In order to have a healthful diet that is balanced and adequate we must become aware of the nutrients our cells need to function properly, and, if necessary, alter our eating habits to fulfill these needs."

"Think about eating and nutrition as behavior that you can control," he writes. "Try to spot deficiencies and, more important, to correct them. And remember, just as mental attitude, hereditary factors and age reflect the performance of your 100 billion cell immune defense army, so does the quality and sufficiency of the nutrients you provide to these vital protectors of your health."

Jane E. Brody wrote in the New York Times on March 21, 1989, "Researchers studying the often surprising effects of nutrition on immunity report that dietary manipulation can become a promising new tool to foster recovery or prevent disease in millions of people."

In her article, Ms. Brody quoted Dr. Robert A. Good, a pediatrician and immunologist at All Childrens Hospital in St. Petersburg, Florida: "We are discovering that some nutrients can be used, not so much as foods, but as moderators, manipulators, or stimulators of the immune system. This could turn out to be pretty powerful medicine if we can understand it better."

According to Ms. Brody, dietary measures might eventually be used to slow the aging of the immune system and to extend the human life-span by delaying the onset of diseases that result from immunological decline. She did not mention shingles but she could have.

In his book "Nutrition and Immunology," Dr. Chandra writes, "Moderation remains the key to a health promoting diet and a healthy immune system."

Dr. Chandra states that nutritional deficiencies and nutritional excesses influence various components of the immune system. "In industrialized nations, immune function has been shown to be compromised in many malnourished hospitalized patients, small-for-gestational age infants, and the elderly. Obesity also may adversely influence immune responses."

According to Dr. Chandra, deficiencies of protein and some amino acids, as well as vitamins A, E, B6 and folate, are associated with reduced immunocompetence. In contrast, excessive intake of fat, in particular polyunsaturated fatty acids, iron, and vitamin E are immunosuppressive. Trace elements modulate immune responses through their critical role in enzyme activity. The role of trace elements in maintenance of immune function and their causal role in secondary immunodeficiency is increasingly being recognized.

Essential nutrients in a healthful diet include carbohydrates, fats, proteins, vitamins and minerals.

Carbohydrates are the main suppliers of fuel to the body's cells. They include starches, sugars and cellulose. Starches are the primary source since they are easily broken down into glucose, the body's primary fuel source, which is carried to cells via the blood stream.

Fats are never water soluble and must be broken down by liver and bile acids before they can enter the system and provide fuel. There are two kinds of fats: saturated such as meat, butter, milk and eggs, which also contain cholesterol; and unsaturated fats such as vegetables, vegetable oils, margarine, and nuts.

Diets high in the kinds of polyunsaturated fatty acids prominent in corn, safflower and soybean oils disrupt the immune system. In excess amounts, these fatty acids delay the maturation of suppressor cells, which act as brakes in the immune system. They also inhibit the formation of lymphocytes, which play a major role in combating disease. Dr. John Kinsella, a biochemist at Cornell University, recommends less consumption of fatty acids and more omega-3 fatty acid as found in fish oil, as well as in many dark-green leafy vegetables.

Proteins provide essential nutrients and raw materials for building the cells that comprise muscle and nerve tissues. Proteins are complex molecules formulated by smaller parts called amino acids. The body is able to produce all the amino acids it needs except for isoleucine, leucine, lysine, methconin, phenylalanine, thrionine, tryptophan and valine. These must be furnished in our diets. Primary sources of proteins are meats, dairy products, fruit and vegetables.

Dr. Maurice E. Shils of the Cornell University Medical College and Dr. Vernon R. Young of the Department of Applied Biological Sciences at the Massachusetts Institute of Technology reported in their 1988 study, "Modern Nutrition in Health and Disease," that severe protein or calorie malnutrition in humans results in marked impairment of both humoral and cell-mediated immune functions.

Drs. Shils and Young point out that diets that provide

a high proportion of protein from animal sources also furnish considerable amounts of saturated fats and cholesterol. They state that the intake of saturated fats and cholesterol from protein foods can be effectively reduced in the following ways:

1. Substitute low-fat or skim milk for whole milk and low-fat cheese for whole-milk cheese.

2. Select only lean cuts of meat and trim off visible fat.

3. Use more poultry, fish, and legumes, and less beef.

4. Restrict the size of portions of meat, poultry and fish to the recommended 4 to 5 ounces daily.

According to Dr. Chandra, deficiencies of protein and some amino acids are associated with reduced immunocompetence.

Arginine, an ordinary component of protein that is available as a concentrated dietary supplement, can stimulate immune function in patients whose immune system is undermined by disease or surgery.

Nucleotides are derived from genetic materials and are present in ordinary diets, but missing from liquid formula diets. Dr. Charles E. Van Buren of the University of Texas and his collaborator, Dr. Fred Rudoph of Rice University, have shown that diets free of nucleotides sharply suppress immune functions.

Vitamins function as catalysts to facilitate the production of energy from nutrients and are generally available in a normal diet.

Deficiency of vitamin A can increase the risk of infections, particularly infections of the eyes and respiratory and gastrointestinal tracts. However, an excess of vitamin A can be toxic, so Dr. Chandra recommends that to avoid an overdose it is best to consume its chemical parent, beta carotene, which is prominent in most dark green and deep-yellow vegetables and fruits. In converting beta-carotene to vitamin A, the body does not produce toxic amounts.

Deficiency of vitamin B6, which occurs among the elderly, impairs cellular immunity and the activity of thymic hormone, which is vital to the maturation of immune cells. Similarly, cellular immunity is depressed by a deficiency of folic acid, a vitamin B needed for cell division.

The B complex vitamins are involved in many aspects of cellular metabolism, including sugar, protein, lipid, and nucleic acid synthesis and degradation, according to Drs. Adrianne Bendich and Marvin Cohen. They wrote in "B Vitamins and Immune Responses," a chapter of Dr. Chandra's book, "Since the cells involved in the generation of both specific and nonspecific immune responses are metabolically active, they would be expected to be affected by B vitamin status. The relationships between reduced intake or deficiency of specific B vitamins and changes in immune function have suggested that immunity can be severely compromised when tissue levels of these vitamins are low or absent.

Each food group makes a special vitamin contribution to the diet. Fruits and vegetables are the principal sources of ascorbic acid; dark green leafy vegetables and deep yellow vegetables and fruits are a major source of carotene; milk is a principal source of riboflavin; meats, poultry and fish are outstanding for niacin, vitamin B6, vitamin B12, and thiamin; and whole-grain and enriched breads and cereals are especially important for thiamin and niacin.

Minerals that are important to the normal functioning of the body include iron, which is needed to carry oxygen throughout the body and to remove carbon dioxide; calcium for building bones and teeth; and zinc for cells that make up your skin. Like vitamins these minerals are not found in the body and must be supplied by the food we eat or food supplements.

Iron deficiency, especially during prenatal and early life, can result in long-term immunological deficiencies that are not correctable by subsequent iron supplements. Iron is a critical ingredient in a number of enzymes that are involved in the killing of infectious organisms.

Selenium is needed for the formation of antibodies and enzymes that take part in immunity. But excessive intake, such as some health-food enthusiasts recommend, can impair immune responses.

Zinc, the most widely studied essential mineral with respect to immunity, is often deficient in diets that derive most of their protein from grains. A low intake of zinc can result in depressed immune responses. Especially at risk are the elderly and people who eat little or no meat and lots of fiber. Zinc is essential to the production of thymic hormones, needed to invigorate the growth of immune cells. Deficiency during prenatal or early life can permanently damage the immune system.

It is believed that zinc may play a special role in the case of shingles. Dr. Patrick O. Tennican, of the Arizona Health Science Center, reports that minute concentration of zinc in cells invaded by herpes viruses caused marked reduction of viral activity without harming uninvaded cells. According to Dr. Richard Passwater, zinc may promote healing by strengthening a cell's integrity and making it more resistant to disease. A word of caution: high levels of zinc can be toxic and should be taken only on the recommendation of a doctor.

In Dr. Chandra's book, Dr. Laurie Hoffman-Goetz contributed a chapter on lymphokines, monokines, and malnutrition. She concludes her chapter with the observaton, "In the past decade there has been a substantial increase in our knowledge about the immune system and the influence of malnutrition on host defense mechanisms. Experimental and clinical studies demonstrate that both macrophage and micronutrient deficiencies modify the development and expression of cellular immune responses."

Dr. Adrianne Bendich summarizes the status of nutritional immunology as follows: "The field of nutritional immunology has evolved from a global view of the effect of generalized malnutrition to determination of the effects of single nutrient deficiencies and now to the point where one has the potential to examine the need for nutrients beyond the level to prevent deficiency. Experiments to determine the nutritional value requirements for optimal immune function need to be encouraged with the understanding that numerous factors including nutrient

interaction, aging, genetic consideration, and environment influences may increase these requirements."

So, we are what we eat, as Lindlahr observed. But
there are other elements that comprise our life-style and
are also essential to an effectively working immune system. We are usually well aware of the need for adequate
sleep. Doctors advise us to get the usual eight hours. Our
mothers tried to instill good sleep habits when we were
young. Employers advise their people that lack of sleep
can affect their job performance and prospects of advancement. Shakespeare's Hamlet ponders its significance in
his famous soliloquy. And yet in the ordering of priorities
how often we fail to recognize that full sleep is absolutely
essential to healthy living and that burning the candle at
both ends can only lead to trouble.

Dr. Hamilton describes the need of sleep as follows:
"During sleep our minds and bodies undergo a form of
rejuvenation. Energy that is spent moving, thinking and
interacting with the external world in our wakeful hours is
turned inward during sleep. Repairs are effected, the
machinery of our bodies is recharged, and our minds get
a needed break as well."

He continues, "Obtaining adequate sleep is very
important for people who have herpes. Too little sleep
deprives your body of the time it needs for physical
reconditioning and has a negative impact on your mental
attitude, leaving you irritable, anxious and poorly pre-
pared to handle the many taxing situations that arise every
day."

There is no general rule for what is an adequate

amount of sleep, for no two systems are exactly alike, and the amount varies as life progresses. The best guide is how you feel afterward. The writer has found that his batteries do not recharge as quickly as when he was a young man and could get along with five or six hours of sleep and mistakenly believed that sleep was a waste of time.

Now, the third factor over which we have some control is the way we live. Our mental attitude, is it positive or negative? How do we handle the usual stresses and can we contain them, reduce them? What feeling do we have about ourselves? Do we have confidence in our ability to cope successfully with life's many problems, including shingles? In his book, "Stress of Life," Dr. H. Selye writes that there is a clear relationship between self-knowledge and therapy. His advice is "know thyself," which essentially is the advice of all psychoanalysts.

Dr. Hamilton emphasizes the relationship between stress and recurrent bouts of shingles. He states that if we accept the proposition that the varicella virus is not completely dormant and is constantly seeking an opportunity to erupt, then stress has a bearing on the time of eruption and helps to explain eruptions that occur in younger people. Dr. Hamilton offers some suggestions for dealing with stress:

"Any alteration in your life—big, small, positive, or negative—can cause stress; the essence of stress is change.

"Many stresses in life can be controlled by anticipating the events that provoke them and by either removing them, changing them, or spacing them out over time. By limiting anticipated stress, unanticipated stress that occasionally occurs may be less damaging.

"Learning to relax, think clearly, and remain calm during unexpected stressful events will help defuse them and diminish their damaging potential.

"The effect of stress can be cumulative. Chronic stress is the most damaging; clusters of stressful events in a short period of time are somewhat less damaging."

Not all medical people agree that stress is a factor. This is probably because stress does not lend itself to a controlled study. There is an unfortunate tendency among many in the medical community to dismiss anecdotal findings, no matter how reasonable they appear to be. The writer's own experience is that controlling stress can moderate the pain of postherpetic neuralgia, but he cannot prove it.

Then there is our physical environment. Do we live in a climate that is constantly testing our ability to survive and if we do and there is no choice, do we dress properly, eat properly, sleep properly? Cold weather does not cause colds, but being cold can diminish our immune capacity and lower our resistance.

For a variety of reasons, we cannot all move to an ideal environment to live. But there is much that we can do to make sure that our environment is not a constant threat to our well-being. Not so long ago we put up with belching smokestacks because we didn't know better. We know better now but there is still a lot of smog and acid rain.

Chapter 12. *Pain*

Pain has intrigued philosophers, theologians, and the medical community for a very long time. It has occupied a significant place in attempts by philosophers to give meaning to man's existence. Pain and pleasure are the opposite poles of life, according to some philosophers such as Bentham, and are the coordinates that measure success, health, and morality.

Pain has played a central role in the religious thought of Western civilization. It has been closely linked with punishment from the very beginning. For her disobedience in the Garden of Eden, Eve was condemned, as stated in Genesis 3:16, to bring forth children in sorrow. The crucifixion and the intense suffering it brought have played a central role in the history of Christianity. The close connection between pain and punishment persisted in the Middle Ages when in Old English and Old French the word for pain was "poena", which was also the word for punishment.

David Bakan writes in "Disease, Pain and Sacrifice", "I regard it as indicative of something important in both the mind of man and the nature of our culture that the dominant image in the history of Western civilization has been one of suffering and pain. It is also noteworthy that in spite of their differences, many of our secular philosophies and our religious traditions should converge in giving pain a central place."

What does this have to do with postherpetic pain? In dealing with pain, it is important to realize that it is not a simple matter like a boil on one's neck but a highly complex experience involving our emotions as well as our body. How we view our pain and rationalize it may determine our success in handling it. Are we being tested for some inexplicable reason? Does our culture, which equates pain with punishment—with incarceration, rejection, execution—suggest that we are doing penance and for what? The very experience of pain, continuing, unrelenting pain, can seriously affect our reasoning and open the door to desperate acts as alternatives. So, pain, any pain, postherpetic pain, is a sensation that involves our psyche, as well as our soma, and in the case of PHN should be dealt with at both levels.

First, let's describe pain in medical terms, not religious, not philosophical. It is a sensory disturbance that is generated in the brain by the receipt of impulses that have traveled to the brain largely along pathways described as the nociceptive system. Throughout the body, on the surface and internally, there are nerve endings, which are the receptors of the nociceptive system. When these nerve endings are stimulated, messages are transmitted to the spinal column and thence to the brain, which may give rise to the experience of pain depending on the interaction of a number of modulating mechanisms.

Describing the pathways of pain in his book, "Therapy of Pain," Dr. Mark Swerdlow states that pain messages are transmitted to the brain through two parallel pathways: one, a rapidly conducting system that feeds into the posterior lateral thalmus and the other a slowly conducting system that feeds into the more central thalmus via a number of relays. Pain impulses reaching the thalmus are relayed to neurons located in the cerebral cortex and now the perception of pain, its severity, and location become apparent to the sufferer.

In most human tissues, nerve fibers are woven like a mesh throughout the tissue. The walls of arteries and veins contain a similar network of nerve fibers that encircle each blood vessel in the form of a sheath. When the nerve fibers are stimulated by mechanical or chemical causes, messages are transmitted through nerve fibers to related peripheral nerves and ultimately to the brain.

Basically, there are two sources of pain, mechanical and chemical. The source of the pain is mechanical when the tissues containing the network of nerve fibers are disrupted by incision, tearing, laceration, or excessive stretching or compression, or when the systems of veins and arteries are affected in the same manner or by marked constriction or dilation of the vessels. Chemical irritation in tissues and blood vessels is the result of high concentrations of one or more of the chemical agents that cause pain: lactic acid, potassium ions, polypeptic kinins, 5-hydroxytryptamine, prostaglandin E, and histamine. Chemicals like lactic acid and potassium ions are released in high concentrations by the cells of anemic tissues, while the other chemical agents are released by cells that have been traumatized and are the major constituents of inflammatory tissues.

It is clear that pain resulting from shingles is the result of chemicals released by cells that have been traumatized and inflamed. In the case of PHN, there are several theories that seek to explain this type of pain. A prominent theory is that the nerve pathways to the spinal cord have been damaged or destroyed by the virus and that as a consequence the normal pain modulating systems are adversely affected, resulting in a flooding of pain impulses to the brain. This is described as deafferentation pain. In other words, the normal afferent pathways do not work and the pain stimuli are exacerbated and detoured to a part of the brain called the medial thalamus. It is explained that the normal pathways do not work because the large nerve fibers have been destroyed, leaving only the small fibers intact. This theoretically could reduce the normal inhibitory effect in transmitting pain information to the dorsal horn, and as a result pain signals become exacerbated.

Other theories attempting to explain PHN pain suggest that the inflammation caused by the virus has not abated, and a third explains that the viral infection continues to rain down the nerve pathways creating pain.

Earlier it was pointed out that the sensation of pain depends on the action of both peripheral and central pain modulating systems along the pathways to the brain. For pain to occur, the messages entering the spinal cord must depolarize the neurons in the spinal nucleus so that they fire up the tracts into the brain. The degree to which depolarization occurs determines the intensity of pain, and so any neurological mechanism that modulates the firing of pain signals will have a significant effect on the experience of pain.

It is believed that depolarization occurs as a result of

the release of a transmitter agent and that this release may be directly influenced by spinal inputs from receptors in the skin, muscles and joint capsules that exert modulating effects on the experience of pain.

This belief has led to the use of tissue massage, manipulation of joints, and the application of tissue vibrators to enhance the discharge from tissue receptors and stimulate the large diameter nerve fibers, and thus diminish the intensity of many kinds of pain.

The writer tried using a vibrator on his forehead to reduce the pain and the numbness with some success. He was not aware of this technique until he was in his third year of PHN. In a period of about two months much of the numbness disappeared and the pain continued to decline.

Dr. Swerdlow points out in his book that the numbness associated with postherpetic neuralgia is the result of selective viral destruction of the dorsal root ganglion cells of the large diameter nerve fibers, which results in the loss of inhibitory effects until receptor neurons regenerate.

He makes the point that increasing age involves progressive degeneration of pain receptors and large diameter nerve fibers throughout the body and this results in the gradual loss of normal central inhibitory effects on the transmission of pain signals and explains the diminished pain tolerance that characterizes middle-aged and elderly people.

In addition to the modulating influences exerted by tissue receptors, pain is also affected by central systems that influence the downward projection of interneurons from the brain stem to the central regions of the mesencephalon and the cerebral cortex. Dr. Swerdlow holds that spinal neurons in the dorsal horn contain high concentrations of enkephalins and that the release of this opiate transmitter, with a chemical structure similar to morphine, is responsible for the diminution of pain. The modulating system discharges continuously throughout life, inhibiting the onward flow of pain impulses from peripheral pain receptors through the spinal cord into the brain.

The effect, according to Dr. Swerdlow, is augmented when one's attention is diverted from the painful site by stimulation elsewhere, or by concentration on some particular task, or when hypnosis is induced. Some drugs such as Valium have the effect of increasing the activity of the neurons that operate this inhibitory system and thereby reduce the pain without affecting the patient's alertness. Apparently, small doses of barbiturates can have an opposite effect when given to patients suffering from chronic pain.

Dr. Benjamin Crue states that the amount of research in the field of centrally acting narcotics and the endorphins and enkephalins is staggering. "It has led," he writes, "to plausible explanations for the long-standing empirical use of analgesic-narcotic combinations."

Using drugs to alleviate pain associated with shingles and PHN is an area where results have been spotty at best. Among the drugs usually used are anti-convulsants (klonopin, tegretol, and dilantin), anti-depressants (doxepin and amitriptyline) and analgesics (aspirin, tylenol) and narcotics. Despite inconclusive showing of these drugs, doctors have no real alternative but to use them and hope that one of them will work effectively.

Studies have shown that electrical or chemical stimulation of neurons in the spinal gray matter inhibits the transmission of pain messages, and that the same effect is achieved with morphine and similar drugs.

Neurons in several regions of the cerebrum are believed to exert modulating influences on the transmission of nerve messages within the spine.

There are other modulating systems, in addition to those mentioned, involving the thalamus, the spinal cord, and the cerebral cortex that block the transmission of pain messages.

A study completed in 1988 by a team headed by Dr. J. Unger of the Department of Neurology at the Technical University of Munich, Germany, disclosed that somatostatin found in the cerbrospinal fluid plays a role in the modification of pain responses. He states, "Opioid peptides are involved in regulation of pain mechanisms but other peptides such as somatostatin may play a role in the modulation of nociceptive responses."

Pain can be influenced in many other ways, by moods, states of anxiety, and by drugs such as benzedrine, marijuana, LSD, and small quantities of alcohol and caffeine, all of which may serve to heighten the perception of pain. To the contrary, tranquility induced by suggestion, hyperventilation, the intake of a large amount of alcohol, and the administration of drugs such as meperidine, can result in reduced cortical activation and diminished pain, according to Dr. Swerdlow.

While the facts about pain transmission and modulation are well known in the medical community, there are different ways of interpreting and applying them. There are two schools of thought concerning chronic pain. The peripheralist believes that chronic pain is the result of some kind of peripheral disturbance and must be treated as such. The centralist takes a different position, that in addition to central pain modulating systems, there are central pain generating mechanisms that apply in the case of most types of chronic pain, except for cancer and arthritis. Dr. Crue, a leading exponent of the centralist concept, believes that centrally generated pain is psychosomatic and should be treated psychiatrically. In his opinion, the view that chronic pain stems from continued nociceptive input "is a widely held medical myth."

Dr. Crue believes that most patients with continuing suffering belong in the category that he describes as "chronic intractable pain" and that these patients, in whom there is no longer any apparent nociceptive input to block or modulate, represent a large group. Patients in this group, after initial beneficial placebo responses wear off, usually experience failure with nerve blocks and chordotomies, according to Dr. Crue. "These are the patients who are costing Americans at least $90 billion a year in lost wages, costly medical care, third-party payments or disability awards in litigation settlements for pain and suffering."

The writer had 10 nerve blocks of the trigeminal nerve over a period of about a month and they had no lasting effect in reducing pain. The pain was eliminated for a period of about three hours, but then it returned and on several occasions with greater intensity.

Dr. Jack J. Pinsky, an associate of Dr. Crue, a member of the New Hope Pain Center, and a supporter of the centralist concept of pain, describes the findings of a study the Center made of the efficacy of its program. "One of our more striking findings is that more than 90% of our patients required no further invasive medical treatment (surgery or nerve blocks) subsequent to their treatment in our Pain Unit. Of interest is the fact that a large percentage (approximately 50%) of our patients received no other (nonsurgical) medical treatment after discharge. This represents a large group in that these patients had a full and lengthy history of having continuously sought many different forms of medical treatment for their problems with chronic pain prior to their treatment at the Pain Unit."

Peripheralists differ with Dr. Crue as to the definition and treatment of chronic pain and to the number of patients who should be placed in this category. It is their position that most pain whether acute or chronic is due to nociceptive input and that those patients who do not fit this definition are few in number.

Dr. Richard H. Morse, director of the Center for Chronic Pain and Disability Rehabilitation, Louisiana State University Medical School, takes the middle road, which he describes as an eclectic stance. He believes that the peripheralist and centralist concepts of pain help to explain different types of pain and are not contradictory.

He has developed a technique for using pain blocks to determine whether pain is central or peripheral. It is based on the theory that the lumbar nerve fibers, which control input of pain impulses to the spinal tract, will react differently depending on the amount of anaesthetic that is injected. Underlying the procedure is the assumption that the smaller and less myelinated fibers will respond first and separately from the larger fibers. A placebo solution of normal saline is used first and if the patient responds with relief, the pain problem is considered psychosomatic. A second solution of very dilute anaesthetic is introduced to block sympathetic fibers without interfering with somatosensory or motor fibers. A positive response is regarded as evidence of sympathetic mediation of pain. A third, more concentrated solution is used to anaesthetize somatosensory fibers, still sparing the largest motor fibers, and here the persistence of pain is indicative of a predominantly central pain mechanism. A fourth and more concentrated solution provides complete motor and sensory paralysis. The failure of pain relief in the face of total peripheral blockade is held as evidence of a central pain mechanism either psychogenic or malingering.

There is some question whether this technique applies in the case of deafferentation pain, that is pain that results from the destruction of nerve pathways and damage to pain modulating mechanisms.

The idea that there is a central pain mechanism would seem to be incontrovertible. How else does one explain the effect that a positive attitude can have on illness? The placebo effect is well known and documented. In almost all trials there is a number of patients who receive useless medication as part of a control group and yet report improvement.

Dr. H. K. Beecher reports in his book, "Disease and the Advancement of Health Science," that he reviewed fourteen studies involving twenty-six groups of patients in which the effect of placebos as pain relievers was studied. The percentages in which relief was obtained varied from 15% to 38%, the median being 35%. Thus, over a wide range of studies, roughly a third of the persons in pain, given a placebo, experienced relief.

The medical community is primarily concerned with pain as a phenomenon associated with the physical body. The person in pain can usually describe its location, its intensity, and, if you ask him if it's physical or psychological, he will quickly respond that it is physical. The possibility that the pain may be psychological makes little sense to the person experiencing it. And the public generally has an aversion to the idea that pain may have its roots in the mind.

But the very fact that pain is an emotional experience indicates that the mind is involved. Pain is a conscious experience. It involves the psyche as well as the body. There are many examples of how the mind can prevail over the body and reduce and even eliminate the sensation of pain. Radical surgery has been performed on people under hypnosis without signs of pain. Counter-irritants, such as intense auditory stimulation, may reduce or abolish pain. Prize fighters, football players, and soldiers in battle may show no signs of pain even when severely injured. The power of auto-suggestion is another example. The writer learned that he could induce a state of tranquility and by suggestion reduce the perception of pain.

A group of investigators from Columbia Presbyterian Medical Center sought to evaluate the effectiveness of psychotherapy in treating disease. One could wish that the disease was postherpetic neuralgia. But, while it concerned patients with ulcerative colitis, their conclusions have application to other diseases such as postherpetic neuralgia. The study involved two groups of patients suffering from colitis for a period of seven years. The groups were matched on the basis of severity of illness, sex, age, and the onset of the disease. One group received psychological therapy, the other did not. Regular examinations were made and systematic ratings of proctoscopic observations and symptoms were recorded. The study concluded, "There is a definite role for psychotherapy in the treatment of ulcerative colitis."

The role of psychiatry in the management of chronic pain has resulted in the development of a team approach to treatment in which the psychiatrist is an integral member. The team concept has resulted in a proliferation of pain centers in the last 25 years. The teams evolved in a number of different directions. Often non-medical members were added, including physical therapists and occupational therapists. In some the emphasis was on the central approach. Most, however, followed the peripheralist concept of treatment.

The earliest pain centers were set up in the 1940s and dealt essentially with nerve blocks. In the 1960s the importance of a multi-disciplined approach became recognized. Two of the pioneers of this approach were Dr.

Benjamin Crue, who founded the Pain Clinic at the City of Hope National Medical Center in Duarte, California, and Dr. John Bonica, who set up a similar facility in Seattle, Washington.

Many of the clinics as they evolved became associated with hospitals, particularly cancer hospitals, universities, and orthopedic and rheumatological centers. The programs of these clinics became multi-disciplinary as more specialists were added to staff first as consultants and then as regular staff.

It is estimated that there are more than 1,000 pain centers and clinics in the United States today. Most centers provide services on both an out-patient and in-patient basis and are staffed with medical and non-medical specialists, including neurosurgeons, neurologists, psychiatrists, anaesthesiologists, and rehabilitation specialists. Unfortunately, there are no published guidelines to assist prospective patients and referring doctors in selecting an appropriate pain center.

Criteria for the management of pain centers and clinics were set up by the Commission on Accreditation of Rehabilitation Facilities of Tucson in 1981. The criteria applied to the manner in which pain centers are operated, not to the kinds of services offered. The criteria were reviewed and adopted by the American Pain Society in 1982 and put into effect by the Commission in 1983. A copy of the criteria can be obtained by writing CARF, 2500 North Pantano Road, Tucson, AZ 85715.

Care should be exercised by postherpetic neuralgia patients in selecting a pain center, since treatment will vary between centers emphasizing a centralist approach and those with a peripheralist pain philosophy.

It should also be determined if the center qualifies for coverage by Medicare and by insurance carriers and whether they accept their payments as payments in full. Some pain centers have had difficulty in the past with Medicare and insurance carriers because of the nature of their services, the type of staff employed, and by problems in demonstrating cost-effectiveness.

Attempts to cut costs and demonstrate cost-effectiveness have resulted in greater emphasis on out-patient services. Dr. Crue says this has led to a general downgrading of new pain teams. "They are now often composed of treaters with fewer years of training and are no longer truly multi-disciplinary. The team leader is often a non-physician (a psychologist, nurse, therapist). The one physician is often a part-time medical director who uses other physicians on an as-needed basis. The psychotherapists are often at a masters degree level, with a part-time psychiatrist as supervisor."

"Thus sadly," Dr. Crue writes, "the future of algology is still in doubt. The pain team movement which has proven medically effective in many patients with chronic pain, when all else has failed, may not be viable in our present socio-economic climate, especially with so much individual patient and collective medical resistance still to be overcome."

Quite possibly Dr. Crue may have overstated his concern, perhaps as a means of challenging his colleagues to push harder for better public understanding.

Chapter 13. *How To Treat Postherpetic Neuralgia*

Treating patients with postherpetic neuralgia has been described as one of the most difficult, challenging, and frustrating tasks facing the medical community. Yet there is no lack of medications and therapies. The problem is that few, if any, function effectively in most cases.

In the pharmaceutical field, the drugs most commonly used are anti-depressants, anti-convulsants, and analgesics.

In 1965 an Australian psychiatrist was the first to recognize that amitriptyline, an anti-depressant, could give relief in truly chronic postherpetic pain problems. He believed that 14 of his patients were depressed, which formed the rationale for using the drug. He achieved good results in 11 of his 14 patients.

It is not difficult to comprehend the effect that any ongoing illness, particularly postherpetic neuralgia, with its unrelenting pain, can have on one's mental state, ranging from down-in-the-dumps to severe anxiety and depression. It has been recognized that depression can have a retarding effect on recovery from illnesses in general. Dr. J. P. Imboden conducted a study in 1961 of a group of patients with undulant fever and found that the amount of time patients continued to manifest symptoms was greater in those who showed signs of depression.

Amitriptyline (Ametril, Elavil, Endep) is widely used in treating postherpetic neuralgia, whether there is evidence of depression or not. It also acts as a mild sedative and usually one tablet at night promises a sound, pleasant night's sleep, without any drugged feeling in the morning. The drug has other properties, which are not fully understood, that have a beneficial effect.

A recent study (1988) by Dr. M. B. Fox and a group of associates showed that of 58 patients with PHN 47% reported moderate or greater relief after a six-week course of treatment with amitriptyline in combination with lorazepam, which compares with 16% for a placebo.

Dr. Russell Portenoy reports that of 23 PHN patients treated with amitriptyline 25% experienced moderate relief after a period of 18 weeks. He points out, however, that the likelihood of a favorable response declines as the duration of PHN increases.

Dr. C. P. N. Watson tested amitriptyline against a placebo in 24 patients who had PHN for more than three months and found a significant improvement in pain moderation.

Other anti-depressants that have been used with moderate success are doxepin and chlorprothixene.

The anti-convulsants (dilantin, tegretol and depakene) are another class of drugs that has been found to be moderately effective in treating PHN. The anti-convulsants were first developed to treat epilepsy. There is no clear understanding of how they work in alleviating PHN pain. Anti-convulsants are usually employed in conjunction with an anti-depressant if a severe lancinating pain is involved. The drug of choice appears to be carbamazepine, although phenytoin, valproate, and clonazepan have also been used. Carbamazepine has particular application in the case of trigeminal neuralgia.

Neuroleptics, such as fluphenazine and haloperidol, have been advocated for PHN in combination with antidepressants, but they have rarely been studied independently. The efficacy of the neuroleptics remains unproved, and their use is limited by the risks of toxicity in elderly patients.

Dr. Crue is a strong believer in the use of narcotics in treating peripheral pain such as shingles, but not in the case of PHN. As a centralist, he questions the use of corticosteroids and analgesics, since, in his view, the pain is not caused by peripheral stimuli but originates in the central nervous system.

Dr. Loeser reports that local infiltration of the painful region with hydrocortisone has been beneficial in a small series of patients, even when this treatment is implemented years after the onset of PHN.

The Department of Neurological Surgery of SUNY Health Science Center undertook a study of the efficacy of aspirin and reported its findings in April 1988. "This simple method of achieving substantial pain control in patients with postherpetic neuralgia has been effective in each of the patients in whom it has been used (the most recent 12 cases have been summarized for this report). It has been more effective than narcotic analgesics, oral anti-inflammatory analgesics, sedatives, tranquilizers, TENS, hypnosis, and the wide variety of operative measures we have tried in the past. Although it was initially used pragmatically, there is now a reasonable rationale for its effectiveness based on more recent insights into the anatomy and neurophysicology of cutaneous nociceptors and the neuropharmacology of aspirin."

A new salve to be applied directly to the affected area was introduced several years ago. Called Zostrix (capsaicin), it was tested by a group of doctors headed by Dr. Joel E. Bernstein of the Department of Dermatology at Northwestern University Medical School, and reported in the Journal of the American Academy of Dermatology in 1987. In an attempt to alleviate the pain of 14 patients with PHN, capsaicin was applied topically to the painful area for a period of four weeks. Of the twelve, nine (75%) experienced substantial relief of their pain. The rationale of the treatment is that the drug, found in the fruits of various specimens of plants of the nightshade family, is known to enhance the release of substance P in the peripheral nerve terminals. Substance P, a neuropeptide, is an important mediator of pain impulses from the periphery to the central nervous system and has been demonstrated in high levels in sensory nerves supplying sites of chronic inflammation.

Another product, Mineral Ice, has been on the market for several years. Its label describes the product as an external pain relieving coolant gel for the temporary relief of minor aches and pains of muscle and joints associated with arthritis, simple backache, strains, bruises, sprains and leg cramps. While PHN is not included, I have used it to relieve the burning pain on my forehead, and prefer it to Zostrix since, if it gets into the eye, it is far less painful than Zostrix. Zostrix, on the other hand, provides more effective and longer relief.

The other approaches that have been followed in seeking to alleviate pain from PHN include anaesthetic, surgical, and neuroaugmentative approaches.

Although anaesthetic techniques have been used often to treat PHN, the evidence of their efficacy is limited to anecdotal reports lacking control and adequate follow-up. Both temporary and neurolytic blocks have been advocated. Dr. Portenoy reports "skin infiltration with local anesthetic alone and repeated peripheral nerve blocks were advocated in one report. Intravenous procaine infusion, administered to a small group of patients, was beneficial in less than half and intravenously administered lidocaine provided only transient relief of painful paroxysms. Sympathetic blockade, used in several large groups of patients, provided temporary relief for less than half. Neurolytic blocks of peripheral nerves have yielded unimpressive results. Two recent reports describe the technique of local cryoanalgesia as applied directly to the painful scars. Results were mixed. The most promising series described partial relief of pain in most treated patients. The use of anesthetic approaches to PHN is therefore not strongly supported."

As already mentioned, I tried blocks of the trigeminal nerve on ten consecutive occasions and did not experience any lasting relief.

Surgical approaches have been tried at every level from skin to cerebrum. Dr. Loeser states "Surgical therapy is warranted only when the patient is disabled by pain. Peripheral neurectomy and doral rhizotomy are of no value. Doral root entry zone lesions may be efficacious.

Thalamic stimulation has also led to excellent pain relief in properly selected patients."

Sir John Watson reports, "Surgical division of sensory nerves or roots and alcohol or phenol injection of the Gasserian ganglion have also been advocated but relief is often temporary."

Dr. Raymond D. Adams in Principles of Neurology, October, 1985, states, "Extensive trigeminal rhizotomy and nucleotomy should be avoided since these surgical measures are not universally successful."

Dr. Portenoy reports, "Neurectomy, rhizotomy, and sympathectomy have been attempted often in the treat- ment of PHN. Occasionally a patient with excellent long-term results has been described, but these approaches are usually unsuccessful. Cordotomy occasionally provides immediate relief of pain, but this is transient and thus the procedure is not recommended. Procedures directed toward brainstem structures, including trigeminal tract- otomy, mesencephalotomy or mesencephalothalamon- tomy and ventrobasal or medial thalamotomy have all provided relief to isolated patients with previously intrac- table PHN. The common recurrence of pain and the potential morbidity involved limits the utility of these op- erations in patients with normal life expectancies; none can be recommended at this time. Topectomy has not been useful and lobotomy or leukotomy, while possibly provid- ing some relief in desperate cases, carries substantial risk to the psychological integrity of the individual."

Dr. Crue's views on the use of surgery are even stronger. "The failures of surgery in dealing with postherpetic neuralgia are well known and notorious," he writes. "They border on malpractice."

A new procedure called dorsal root entry zone lesions may prove effective, but too few cases have been reported to permit any kind of conclusion. Drs. A. H. Friedman and B. S. Nashold described good results in fourteen out of seventeen patients who underwent this procedure.

Another technique involves stimulation in an attempt to activate endogenous pain-modulating systems. They include counter-irritation, TENS, acupuncture, dorsal column stimulation and deep brain stimulation.

The application of a small hand vibrator to the affected area together with an ethyl chloride spray is a common technique. In a study of eighty-six patients, Dr. E. M. Todd reported in 1965 that "relief is occasionally dramatic after the first few treatments, but in most instances improvement is less spectacular. The usual course is one of rather gratifying initial improvement with slow irregular progress thereafter."

Dr. D. Taverner reported in Lancet in 1960 that in a group of sixteen patients with well-established PHN, twelve obtained partial relief with repeated application of ethyl chloride spray alone.

Considerable experience has been had with transcutaneous electrical nerve stimulation (TENS) over the last dozen years. The procedure involves applying low voltage electrical shocks to the affected nerve when pain erupts. Generally, the experience is nonpainful and tingling. Pain relief often outlasts stimulation by hours. Dr.

P. W. Nathan reports that thirteen of thirty patients with longstanding PHN achieved moderate to complete relief by using the stimulator as needed. Analgesia outlasted stimulation by many hours in ten patients, and although follow-up data was incomplete, a majority of patients appeared to benefit for some time. Results from other studies have been generally inconclusive. Dr. Anne Gershon found that the intermittent use of TENS was unsuccessful in seventeen patients with chronic PHN.

Acupuncture has been tried but usually unsuccessfully. Dr. G. T. Lewith found that acupuncture was of little value when compared with placebo in sixty-two patients.

Deep brain stimulation was attempted by Dr. J. Siegfried in a group of ten patients with longstanding trigeminal PHN. Eight obtained good to excellent relief that lasted seven to seventeen months of follow-up. A study by Dr. G. L. Mazars reported complete analgesia in five of eleven patients.

A new technique involves the use of lasers. A German group of doctors, headed by Dr. R. Brunner of the Department of Dermatology of the University of Munich treated twenty-eight patients with chronic PHN using a krypton laser, of whom sixteen experienced a marked reduction or complete cessation of pain. Dr. Brunner offers the following rationale for this procedure: "It may be that the polarized laser light influences the bipolar phospholipids of the cell membrane. In addition, a direct influence on the metabolism of various mediators of inflammation seems possible."

Many avenues of approach are being explored to find

better ways of dealing with PHN. Completely different from any others cited thus far is one pursued by Drs. Shuster, E. Tunks, and L. Stitt, members of the faculty of Health Sciences of McMaster University, Canada. They conducted a study of eleven subjects experiencing chronic pain who participated in a six-week exercise program. Subjective pain, state of anxiety, and mechanical pain threshold changes were measured before and after exercise and control periods. Cardiovascular fitness, attitudes towards exercise, and coping skills were evaluated at the beginning and end of the six-week exercise period. A significant difference in anxiety was observed during the exercise sessions as well as in control periods. Changes in the subjects' beliefs about exercise and use of coping skills during exercise were significant. The study concludes that exercise can have a positive long-term psychological effect on ability to cope with chronic pain.

Dr. Benjamin Crue has a four prong approach to dealing with PHN. The first three we have already discussed, i.e., anti-depressants, anti-convulsants, counterirritation therapy. The fourth he considers of equal importance and that is what he calls the laying on of hands. He explains that the support of family and friends is essential for an individual to be able to cope successfully with pain.

As stated earlier, treatment of PHN appears to be directed entirely at dealing with the associated pain and not with the condition itself. Apparently, it is presumed that the damaged nerve pathways, pain modulating systems, and nerve endings will in time restore themselves, without the benefit of medication.

REPORTED TREATMENTS FOR POSTHERPETIC NEURALGIA

Pharmacologic

Non-narcotic analgesics
Narcotic analgesics
Anticonvulsants
Tricyclic antidepressants
Phenothiazines
Vitamins E, B 12
Corticosteroids
Intravenous procaine
Levodopa
Ergot derivatives
Protamine
Pimozide
Baclofen

Anaesthetic

Local infiltration
Peripheral nerve block
Epidural block
Sympathetic block

Surgical

Undermining or excising skin
Cryoprobe nerve lesions
Peripheral neurectomy
Dorsal rhizotomy
Sympathectomy
Dorsal root entry zone lesions
Cordotomy
Trigeminal tractotomy
Cingulumotomy
Frontal lobotomy
Thalamic stimulation

Other

Diathermy
Vibration
Ultrasound
Acupuncture
Transcutaneous electric stiumulation
Ethyl chloride spray

Herpes Zoster and Postherpetic Neuralgia, Dr. John D. Loeser, University of Washington, Published by Elsevier Science Publishers, 1986

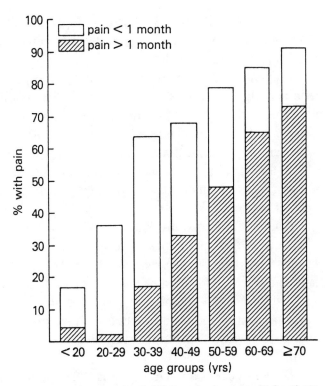

The prevalence and duration of pain among 916 patients with zoster, by age. Modified with permission from de Moragas and associates (68).

From Annals of Internal Medicine, Vol. 108, No. 2, February 1988, by Dr. Stephen Straus, National Institutes of Health.

Chapter 14. *Can Postherpetic Neuralgia Be Prevented?*

Applying a line from Shakespeare to the prevention of postherpetic neuralgia, one could say "tis a consummation devoutedly to be wished."

Preventing shingles from developing into postherpetic neuralgia continues to baffle the medical community. It is generally conceded that a better understanding of the pathology of PHN is required before effective ways of preventing it can be developed.

In the meantime, studies are examining the efficacy of corticosteroids and antiviral medications singly and together to prevent PHN.

A number of uncontrolled studies of small numbers of patients with acute herpes zoster treated with corticosteroids have demonstrated a preventive effect. Dr. W. H. Eaglstein treated 10 patients over 60 years of age with a corticosteroid and a control group of 15 with a placebo. Thirty percent of the group treated with steroids developed PHN, which compares with 73% in the placebo group.

Dr. K. Keczkes and Dr. A. M. Basheer undertook a study comparing steroids with carbamazepine. They found that 65% of the 20 patients in the carbamazepine group developed PHN lasting two or more months, while only 30% of the 10 patients in the steroid group developed PHN.

The rationale for steroid use, according to Dr. Straus, is to limit inflammation and subsequent scarring in the dorsal root ganglia, factors that might be responsible for chronic pain.

In a study of 130 patients with acute zoster, Drs. S. Harvery Sklar and J. S. Wigand in 1985 were able to demonstrate that early treatment of shingles with adenosine monophosphate effectively suppressed postherpetic neuralgia. Twelve subjects experienced some residual discomfort that eventually cleared and the balance escaped PHN. No recurrence of pain was reported by any patient two years after therapy.

A group of doctors headed by Dr. P. Duschet of the Department of Dermatology at the Hospital Vienna Lainz, Austria, tested alpha interferon and acyclovir in a group of 127 patients and found that neither prevented PHN.

Dr. A. Colding reported in 1969 that sympathetic blockade with a local anaesthetic in acute herpes zoster markedly reduced the incidence of PHN. Although he treated a large number of patients in this fashion, his work was uncontrolled and a substantial number of patients were unavailable for follow-up.

A letter from Dr. Joan Drucker of the Department of Clinical Microbiology and Immunology of Burroughs Wellcome summarizes the current situation in the following way: "Preventing herpes zoster from causing postherpetic neuralgia would be a great discovery. The pathogenesis of postherpetic neuralgia is still poorly understood. There is controversy whether the pain is caused by viral damage or the inflammatory response to infection. Both antiviral and anti-inflammatory drugs have been tried, without clearcut success. One study of acyclovir suggested that patients treated within 72 hours of the appearance of the rash had a lower incidence of postherpetic neuralgia. Another study showed that acyclovir has no benefit when PHN is already established. We expect to conduct further research in this area. The National Institutes of Health is currently sponsoring a clinical trial to elucidate the answer. The results are still more than a year away. Until more is known about the underlying causes of postherpetic neuralgia, it will be difficult to target specific therapy."

Chapter 15. *A Summing Up*

In putting this book together, the writer made several assumptions.

One, that the reader has shingles and that he would like to know what it is all about and whether he or she is being treated properly and how complications like postherpetic neuralgia can be avoided.

Two, he already has postherpetic neuralgia and would like to know what he can do to hasten recovery.

Three, he has had shingles and postherpetic neuralgia and would like to know if a recurrence can be prevented and how.

Four, the family and friends of the sufferer would like to know what shingles and PHN are all about and what they can do to help.

Five, he may be a member of the medical community and would like to have access to the information that I have collected.

With these assumptions in mind, the writer would like to summarize the highlights of the information that has been presented.

1. Shingles is nothing to trifle with. It can have very serious complications, so get to a doctor at once. Your chances of quick recovery and avoidance of PHN and other complications are best if antiviral treatment is started within 72 hours of the first signs of shingles.

2. A dermatologist or an internist are best qualified to help you. A neurologist is usually not involved until shingles has developed into postherpetic neuralgia.

3. Follow your doctor's advice to the letter, but be sure that he is qualified. If he thinks the best way of dealing with shingles is to let it run its course, quickly find another and more experienced doctor.

4. You are not unique in being infected. The disease has been around for a very long time, probably since the beginning of time, and has infected people in all walks of life. Well over a million people are infected annually. It has nothing to do with promiscuity, as other forms of herpes imply.

5. It is not a forerunner of cancer.

6. The culprit in the picture is the varicella virus which you acquired when you had chickenpox as a child and which has resided in your system ever since waiting for a chance to break out.

7. The varicella zoster virus has broken out in your case and caused shingles because your immune system has been impaired for one or more of the following reasons: age, past cancer, the use of chemotherapy and radiation, immune suppressive drugs such as steroids, transplants, trauma, unusual stress.

8. The drug of choice in dealing with shingles is acyclovir either by itself or in conjunction with a cortico-steroid.

9. There are non-medical things that you can do to speed recovery. For example: lots of rest, moderate exercise, and avoidance of stress.

10. You can help ameliorate the pain with icepacks, a hand vibrator, and the application of Zostrix and Mineral Ice.

11. A balanced diet is very important, with emphasis on foods and supplements that can enhance your immune system.

12. Your life-style is important. Settle for a life-style where the emphasis is on health, moderation, and the absence of stress.

13. How you deal with your infection and what you do to strengthen your immune system can affect the possibility of a second or third attack of shingles.

14. A vaccine to prevent chickenpox in children will become available some time in 1990 and may end the threat of shingles for that generation. Licensing its use to prevent shingles among adults probably won't occur for several years. Timing could be accelerated if public pressure were exerted on Congress and the Administration.

15. It is very, very important that you do not allow this nasty infection to take over your life, which is a real possibility if recovery drags out for a long time. You need to be actively engaged in activities, like a hobby, that will divert your attention from the pain. Family understanding and support are essential.

16. Exercise on a regular basis is very important. Nothing strenuous like running. Long comfortable walks are fine.

17. There are many pain centers across the country that are designed to help you with the pain of postherpetic neuralgia. But be careful in your selection, for their methods differ widely, and some are less reliable than others. Your doctor should be able to help you select the

right one.

18. The drugs used most frequently in dealing with PHN are anti-depressants, anti-convulsants and analgesics. Their success ratio is spotty. More research into the pathogenesis of PHN is necessary before real progress can be made in finding an effective remedy.

19. Not all doctors have had broad experience in dealing with shingles and PHN. A survey of internists, dermatologists and neurologists undertaken by the writer disclosed limited knowledge of the therapies being used to deal with the infections. So, it is very important that you find a doctor who has the necessary credentials to treat you properly.

20. One last suggestion, take a positive attitude. Tell yourself over and over again that this too will pass. And it will.

Good luck.

Post Script

When you consider that 1.2 million people suffer from shingles annually, that over the next twenty years about 24 million people will experience the agony of shingles, that over the course of a lifetime one out of five will be affected, that annually over 100 thousand endure the indescribable pain of postherpetic neuralgia for anywhere from a few months to as long as twenty years and that for some suicide is chosen as a last-resort alternative, it is amazing that the disease does not occupy a higher priority in the medical community. It is time for change. It is time for pressure to be placed on government health services to devote more time, thought, energy and funding to ending the misery that plagues so many people, particularly those fifty years and older, our senior citizens who are senior not only in years but in neglect. Other diseases like cancer, heart disease, and Alzheimers have their well organized and well funded spokes-organizations to plead their cases, but shingles and postherpetic neuralgia have none. Is it not time that you, the afflicted, a relative of the afflicted, or just a concerned friend, petition your Congressmen, the Administration, your state and community representatives, and organizations like AARP to exert the pressure that is needed to wake up the medical community to action?

The chickenpox vaccine, when it becomes available, may end the threat of shingles for the newborn and application of the vaccine to adults, which is several years away at least, may write finis to the disease for many in their middle-years. But the great need now and for some years to come is finding effective means of moderating the disease, keeping it from developing into postherpetic neuralgia, and accelerating recovery when it develops into postherpetic neuralgia. One of the doctors that the writer interviewed described shingles as "one of the most difficult, distressing and frustrating problems in modern medicine." Question: Does this have to continue?

Glossary

Acyclovir. An antiviral drug that is available under the trade name Zovirax in oral, intravenous, and topical forms. It is particularly effective when administered very soon after the shingles symptoms erupt, preferably within 72 hours. The drug blocks the replication of the varicella zoster virus.

Adenine arabinoside. An antiviral agent (trade name, Vidarbine) that has been used effectively in treating shingles.

Adenosine monophosphate. A combination of adenosine and phosphoric acid. It belongs to the family of nucleotides, which are the basic structural units of DNA and RNA.

Adrenocorticotropic hormone. Affects the growth and activity of the outer portion of the adrenal gland, which lies near the kidney. The adrenal gland produces steroids like sex hormones, adrenalin, and hormones that are concerned with metabolic functions.

Afferent fibers. Nerve fibers bringing pain impulses from the pain receptors in the body to the central nervous system.

Amantadine hydrochloride. Has pharmacological actions as both an anti-Parkinsons drug and an antiviral drug. It appears to prevent the release of infectious viral nucleic acid into the host cell.

Amitriptyline. An anti-depressant, with mild tranquilizing properties, used in ameliorating the pain of PHN.

Antigen. Various materials such as microorganisms, foreign proteins, toxides that induce a state of sensitivity and resistance and stimulate the production of antibodies.

Autohemotherapy. A means of treating disease by withdrawing and re-injecting a patient's own blood.

Clonazepan (Klonopin). An anti-convulsant useful in the treatment of PHN and seizures.

Codon. A triplicate of nucleotides that is part of the genetic code and provides genetic code information for the production of specific amino acids.

Carbamazepine. An anti-convulsant used to control the paroxymal, lancinating pain in PHN.

Corticosteroid. A steroid that has similar properties to the steroid hormone produced by the adrenal cortex. It is used to alter and heighten immune responses to shingles.

Cytosine arabinoside. A chemotherapeutic agent with antiviral inhibiting properties that inhibits the biosynthesis of DNA.

Darvon. A mild narcotic analgesic structurally related to methadone. Used for the relief of mild to moderate pain.

Deafferentation. Loss of sensory nerve fibers.

Dermatome. An area of skin that is supplied by an afferent nerve fiber from a single dorsal ganglion along the spine.

Deoxyribose. A pentose sugar that is a structural element of DNA.

Depakene. An anti-epileptic agent, used in the treatment of petit mal, PHN, and complex seizures.

Dilantin. An anti-epileptic drug used to control PHN and seizures.

Dimethyl sulfoxide. A penetrating solvent that enhances the absorption of therapeutic agents through the skin and is used as an analgesic and an antinflammatory agent.

Disseminated zoster. This describes zoster that has spread beyond the original dermatome to other parts of the body.

DNA. The auto-reproducing component of chromosomes and viruses and the repository of heredity characteristics. It is made of two strands, each consisting of four nucleotides; adenine, thymine, guanine and cystine.

Doxepin. An anti-depressant for the relief of depression and pain.

Dorsal root. One of a pair of nerve roots, flanking the spinal cord and consisting of sensory fibers, that convey pain impulses to the spinal cord.

Elavil (Amitriptyline). An anti-depressant with sedative effects.

Encephalon. That portion of the cerebrospinal axis contained within the cranium.

Encephalitis. Inflammation of the brain.

Encephalotomy. Dissection or incision of the brain.

Endep. An anti-depressant.

Endorphins. An endogenous brain substance (polypeptide) that binds to opiate receptors in various areas of the brain and thereby raises the pain threshold.

Enkephalin. Naturally occuring pentapeptides that have potent opiate-like effects and serve as neurotransmitters. Classified as endorphins, they occur in nerve endings of brain tissue, spinal cord and the gastrointestinal tract.

Fluoro 5 iodarabinosylcytosine (FIAC). An antiviral agent that is particularly effective when administered to immune suppressed individuals.

Folic acid. An acid that stimulates the production of leukocytes which play an important role in the immune system.

Gamma globulin. A class of proteins that contain antibodies.

Ganglion. Located in pairs along the spinal cord, it is an aggregation of nerve cell bodies that transfer nerve impulses from nerve fibers to the spinal cord.

Genome. Total gene complement of a set of chromosomes. The genome of varicella virus contains 70 genes distributed about equally between two DNA strands.

Glaucoma. A disease of the eye characterized by increased pressure within the eyeball and gradual loss of vision.

Glycoprotein. Consists of a compound of protein with a carbohydrate group.

Griseofulvin. An antibiotic used as an antifungal in the treatment of dermatophytic infections.

Histamine. A compound that is responsible for the dilation and increased permeability of blood vessels which play a role in allergic reactions.

Hydrocortisone. A corticosteroid used to treat inflammation.

5 hydroxytryptamine. Believed to be a neurotransmitter of pain in the brain.

Idoxuridine. An antiviral drug used to diminish pain.

Imipramine hydrochloride. An anti-depressant used to treat depressive illnesses and to relieve the anxiety and nervousness that may accompany these problems.

Interferon. A substance produced in cell tissues in response to infection by viruses, capable of inducing a state of resistance to the infection.

Iridocyclitis. Inflammation of the iris of the eye and eyebrows.

Keratitis. Inflammation of the cornea.

Kinin. One of a number of substances having pronounced and dramatic effects on pain transmission. Some are pain regulators, others cause contraction of smooth muscle and hypertension and have become important in dealing with inflammation and shock.

Klonopin. An anti-convulsant used to control PHN pain.

Lobotomy. Severance of nerve fibers by incision into the brain to relieve pain.

Lactic acid. Used internally to prevent gastrointestinal fermentation.

Leukocyte. White blood cells belonging to the myeloid, lymphoid and monocyclic categories. Included in the myeloid group are granulocytes, which include neutrophils, eosinophils, and basophils, important elements of the immune system.

Leukotomy. An operation that involves cutting the white matter of the frontal lobe of the brain to reduce pain.

Lioresal. A muscle relaxant and antispastic used for the relief of spasms and pain. ˡ

Lipids. Together with proteins and carbohydrates constitute the principal structural components of living cells.

Lymphocytes. Lymph cells, which are white blood cells, are formed in lymphoid tissue throughout the body.

Lymphokinesis. The circulation of lymph cells in the lymphatic vessels.

Macrophages. Large phagocytes, which are present in the linings of various organs and tissues, and are part of the immune system's defenses.

Mesencephalon. The midbrain.

Mesenchephalotomy. The sectioning of any structure in the midbrain, especially of the spinthalamic tracts for the relief of severe pain.

Monocytes. A relatively large mononuclear leukocyte (white blood cell) normally found in lymph nodes, spleen, bone marrow, and connective tissues.

Myelin. A mixture of lipids (cholesterol, phospholipids, sphisngolipids, phosplictides and plasmalogens) and protein material arranged in layers around nerve fibers.

Myelitis. Inflammation of the spinal cord or bone marrow.

Myocardial infarction. Death of tissue around the middle layer of the heart, resulting from the arrest of blood circulation in the artery.

Neuropeptides. Believed to act as transmitters of pain and includes enkephalins and endophins.

Nucleotide. A combination of nucleic acid, purine, sugar and phosphate. It is part of the basic structure of DNA and RNA.

Necrosis. Death of one or more cells or a portion of tissue or organ, resulting in irreversible damage.

Neurectomy. Excision of a segment of a nerve.

Neutrophils. A mature white blood cell in the granulocytic series, formed in the bone marrow.

Nociceptive system. A complex of pathways by which pain is transmitted from nerve endings in the body to the central cortex.

Pathogenesis. Origination and development of a disease.

Pathology. Study of the essential nature of a disease and of structural and the functional changes proceeded by the disease.

Peptide. A compound of several amino acids. Polypeptide is formed by the union of a number of amino acids.

Percocet. A semi-synthetic narcotic analgesic for the relief of moderate to moderately severe pain.

Prednisone. A corticosteroid for the relief of pain due to inflammation. It is also immunosuppressive.

Prostaglandins. A class of physiologically active susbtances present in many tissues that perform a variety of hormone-like actions, as in controlling blood pressure and smooth muscle contractions.

Rhizotomy. Cutting the anterior or posterior spinal nerve roots for the relief of pain.

RNA. (ribonucleic acid) A polynucleotide found in all cells in both nuclei and cytoplasm, and in many viruses, and serves as a messenger for DNA codes in producing amino acids.

Scleritis. Hardening of nervous tissues and fibers, resulting from chronic inflammation.

Selenium. A metallic element similar to sulphur.

Soma. The body including the head and neck, without the limbs.

Sympathectomy. Excision of a segment of a sympathetic nerve or ganglion.

Thalamotomy. Excising a selected portion of the thalmus.

Tegretol. (carbamazepine) Is used as an anti-convulsant, particularly in connection with trigeminal neuralgia.

Topectomy. Removal of specific portion of the cervical cortex.

Triamcinolone. A glucocorticoid used as an anti-inflammatory.

Zostrix. (capsaicin) A plant derivative that alters neuropeptide concentrations in certain nerves and reduces pain.

Bibliography

Dr. Raymond D. Adams
Massachusetts General Hospital
Principles of Neurology
McGraw Hill 1985

David Bakan
Disease, Pain and Sacrifice
University of Chicago Press, 1968

Dr. Henry Balfour
University of Minnesota Health Sciences Center
Shingles: Seeds of Fire
University of Minnesota Press, 1984
Varicella Zoster Virus Infections in Immunocompromised Host
American Journal of Medicine, Vol .85, 2A, 1988

Charles Baudouin
Suggestion and Autosuggestion
George Allen Ltd.
London, England, 1920

Dr. B. Barker Beeson
Autohemotherapy in the Treatment of Herpes Zoster
Archives of Dermatology, 1922

Dr. Joel E. Bernstein
Northwestern University Medical School
Treatment of Chronic Postherpetic Neuralgia
Journal of the American Academy of Dermatology 1987

Dr. A. Bouckoms
Massachusetts General Hospital
Intravenous Lorazepam for Pain Relief of Postherpetic Neuralgia
Fifth World Congress on Pain
Hamburg, Germany, August 1987
Elsevier Science Publishers

Dr. R. Brunner
Department of Neurology
University of Munich, Germany
Applications of Laser Light
Current Problems in Dermatology, Vol. 15

Dr. Frank Bucci, Jr.
Albany Medical College of Union University Albany, NY
Dr. Robert A. Schwarz
University of Medicine, New Jersey Medical School, Newark, NJ
Neurological Complications of Herpes Zoster
American Family Physician, 1988

Dr. Ranjit Kumar Chandra
Departments of Pediatrics, Medicine and Biochemistry
Memorial University Hospital of Newfoundland,
St. John's, Newfoundland, Canada.
Nutrition and Immunology
Alan R. Liss, Inc., 1988
Hoffman LaRoche Award Lecture of the Canadian Society for
Nutritional Sciences,
The Lancet, March 26, 1983.
Golan Memorial Lecture
Northshore University Hospital
Cornell University Medical College,
New York, February 13, 1985
Journal of Pediatric Gastroenterology and Nutrition
Raven Press, New York

Dr. W. Christe
Free University of Berlin, Germany
Effect of Early Intravenous Acyclovir
Clinical Journal of Pain, Vol. 4 ,No. 2, 1988

Dr. Benjamin L. Crue, Jr.
Medical Director
Durango Pain Rehabilitation Center,
Durango, Colorado

Emeritus Clinical Professor of Neurological Surgery
University of Southern California School of Medicine
Los Angeles, California
Neuritis, Neuropahy and Neuralgia
Current Concepts in Pain
Vol. 1, No. 6, 1983
Painful Neuropathies and Nerve Root Lesions and Syndromes
Handbook of Chronic Pain Management, 1988

Philip Marshall Dale
Medicial Biographies,
University of Oklahoma Press, 1952

Drs. Andrew J. Davison and James E. Scott
Institute of Virology,
Glascow, Scotland
DNA Sequence of Varicella Zoster Virus
National Institutes of Health, 1986

Fighting Disease
Prevention Magazine
Rodale Press, Pennsylvania

Dr. Richard Dobson
Editor
American Academy of Dermatology
Preventing Postherpetic Neuralgia
Journal of the American Academy of Dermatology

Dr. P. Duschet
Department of Neurology
Hospital Vienna Lainz, Austria
Treatment of Herpes Zoster on Recombinant Alpha Interferon vs
Acyclovir
International Journal of Dermatology, April, 1988

Sir William Fergusson
Notes and Reflections of a Professional Life
Longman Press, London, 1846

Dr. Reuben Friedman
Emperors Itch,
Froben Press, 1940

Dr. A. E. Friedman-Kein
NYU Medical Center
Herpes Zoster: A Possible Early Clinical Sign for Development of
AIDS in High Risk Individuals
Journal of American Academy of Dermatology, 1985

The New Human Genetics
National Institute of General Medical Science
US Department of Health and Human Services
NIH Publication No. 84-662, September 1984

Stop that Germ
Time Magazine, May 23, 1988

Drs. Charles Grose and Roger H. Geller
University of Iowa, College of Medicine
Varicella Zoster Virus Infection and Immunization in the Healthy
and the Immunocompromised Host
CRC Critical Reviews in Oncology/Hematology
Vo. 8, Issue 1, 1988

Dr. Richard Hamilton
The Herpes Book
J. P. Farcher, 1980

Dr. A. R. Hayward
University of Colorado School of Medicine
Cellular Interactions in the Lysis of Varicella Zoster Virus Infected
Human Fibroblasts
Clinical Immunology, 1986

Lysis of Varicella Zoster Virus Infected B Lymphoblasts by
Human T. Cells,
Journal of Virology, April, 1986

Dr. K. Higa
School of Medicine, Fukuoka University, Japan
Implications of Antibodies to VZV in Herpetic Pain
Fifth World Conference on Pain,
Hamburg, Germany, August, 1987
Elsevier Science Publishers

Dr. R. Edgar Hope-Simpson
Epidemeological Research Unit
Cirencester, England
Nature of Herpes Zoster; Long Term Study and New Hypothesis
Proceedings Royal Society of Medicine, 58, 9-20, 1965

Dr. Anne Gershon
Columbia University College of Physicians and Surgeons
Risk of Zoster after Varicella Vaccination
New England Journal of Medicine, March 3, 1988

Dr. J. C. Huff
University of Colorado School of Medicine
Antiviral Treatment in Chickenpox and Herpes Zoster
Journal of American Academy of Dermatology
Vol. 12, No. 1, 1988
Therapy of Herpes Zoster with Oral Acyclovir
American Journal of Medicine,
Vol. 85, No. 2A, 1985

Book of Job
Old Testament

Dr. B. E. Juel-Jensen
Treatment of Zoster with Idoxuridine in Dimethyl Sulphoxide
British Medical Journal, Vol. 4, 1970

Dr. R. B. King
Department of Neurological Surgery
SUNY Health Science Center
Management of Pain Associated with Herpes Zoster and
Postherpetic Neuralgia
Pain, April 1988

Dr. S. Lawrence Kruger and John Liebeskind
Neural Mechanisms of Pain
Raven Press, 1984

Dr. Charles Lampton
DNA and the Creation of Life
Arco Publishing Co., 1983

Dr. Robert Lawrence
NYU Medical Center
Risk of Zoster After Varicella Vaccination
New England Journal of Medicine, March 3, 1988

Dr. Brian Leland-Jones
Memorial Sloan Kettering Hospital
Fluoro 5 — Idoarabinosylcytosine, New Potent Viral Agent
Journal of Infectious Diseases, Vol. 154, No. 3, 1986

Drs. Myron J. Levin and Brenda J. Hershey
Dana Farber Cancer Institute
Drs. John A. Zaia and Gayle Robinson
City of Hope Medical Center, California
Dr. L. Gray Davis of Wellcome Research Laboratories, North
Carolina
Topical Acyclovir Treatment of Herpes Zoster in Immunocompro-
mised Patients
American Academy of Dermatology, Vol. 13, No 4, 1985

Dr. John D. Loeser
Department of Neurological Surgery
University of Washington

Herpes Zoster and Postherpetic Neuralgia
Elsevier Science Publishers, 1986

Dr. Joseph Melnick
Baylor University
Herpes Zoster
Review of Microbiology, 1987

Dr. Quentin N. Myrik
Nutrition and Immunology
Chapter 32
Modern Nutrition in Health and Disease
Lea & Febiger, 1988

Dr. Michael Oxman
Dermatology in General Medicine
McGraw Hill, September, 1986

Dr. Gerald L. Mandell
Principles and Practices of Infectious Disease
John Wiley & Sons, New York, 1987

Dr. M. B. Max
National Institutes of Health
Amitriptyline but not Lorazepam Relieves PHN
Neurology, Vol. 38, 1988

Drs. Jeffrey M. Ostrove and Genevieve Inchausepe
National Institutes of Health
Biology of Varicella Zoster Virus
Published by NIH

Drs. Russell K. Portenoy, Christopher Dumas, and Kathleen Foley
Memorial Sloan Kettering Hospital, New York
Acute Herpetic and Postherpetic Neuralgia: Clinical Review and
Current Management
Annals of Neurology, Vol. 20, No. 6, 1986

Drs. Barbara T. Post and John T. Philbrick
Department of Medicine, University of Virginia
Do Corticosteroids Prevent PHN?: A Review
Journal of American Academy of Dermatology, March, 1988

Dr. W. H. Prusoff
Yale University School of Medicine
Idoxuridine
Martinus Nijhoff Publishing, 1988

Dr. M. W. Ragozzino
Mayo Clinic
Population Based Study of Herpes Zoster and Its Sequelae
Medicine, 1982

Drs. M. W. Ragozzino and L. Kurland
Subsequent Risk of Rheumatoid Arthritis in Patients Diagnosed
With Herpes Zoster
Lancet 2{8303} :884, 1982

Drs. M. W. Ragozzino, L. Kurland, and L. Melton
Epidemiological Investigation of the Association Between Herpes
Zoster and Multiple Sclerosis
Neurology 33:648-649, 1983

Drs. M. W. Ragozzino, L. Melton, L. Kurland and C. Chu
Herpes Zoster and Diabetes Mellitus; An Epidemiological Investi-
gation
Journal Chronic Diseases 36:501-505, 1983

Drs. M. L. Ragozzino and L. Kurland
Investigation of the Association Between Herpes Zoster and
Parkinson's Disease
Neuroepidemiology 2:89-92, 1983

Dr. Victor Robinson
Essay on the History of Medicine
Memorial Volume
Froben Press, 1948

A. L. Rowse
Biography of Jonathon Swift
Charles Scribner Sons, 1975

Arthur Rubenstein
My Many Years
Knopf, 1980

Dr. Mark H. Sawyer
National Institute of Allergy & Infectious Diseases
Treatment and Prevention of Varicella Zoster
Annual Internal Medicine, 1988

Drs. M. Schuster, E. Tunks and L. Stitt
Health Sciences, McMaster University
Hamilton, Ontario, Canada
Short Term Effects of Exercise on Chronic Pain
Fifth World Congress on Pain, Hamburg, Germany
August 1987,
Elsevier Science Publishers

Dr. Robert A. Schwartz
University of Medicine of the New Jersey Medical School,
Newark, NJ
Neurological Complications of Herpes Zoster
American Family Physician, 1988

Dr. D. H. Shepp
Fred Hutchinson Cancer Research Center
Seattle, Washington
Current Therapy of Varicella Zoster
American Journal of Medicine, Vol. 85, 2A, 1988

Dr. Maurice E. Shils
Professor Emeritus of Medicine, Cornell University Medical
College
Dr. Vernon R. Young
Professor of Nutritional Biochemistry

Department of Applied Biological Science
Massachusetts Institute of Technology
Modern Nutrition in Health and Disease
Lea & Febiger, Philadelphia, 1988

Dr. J. Harvey Sklar
Shingles Clinic
Englewood Hospital, New Jersey
Treatment and Prevention of Neuralgia with Adenosine Mono-
phosphate
Journal of American Medical Association, Vol. 253, 10, 1985

Irwin Stone
The Healing Factor; Vitamin C
Grosset Dunlap, 1972

Drs. Nigel D. Stow and Andrew J. Davison
Research Council, Virology Unit,
Institute of Virology, Glascow
Identification of Varicella Zoster Virus Origin of DNA Replication
Glascow, 1986
Published by NIH, 1986

Dr. Stephen Straus
National Institutes of Health
Bethesda, Maryland
Varicella Zoster Virus Infections
Annals of Internal Medicine, Vol. 108, No. 2, 1988
Structure of Varicella Zoster Virus DNA
Published by NIH, 1981

Dr. William H. Sweet
Massachusetts General Hospital
Deafferentation Pain
Neurosurgery Vol. 15, No. 6, 1984

Dr. Mark Swerdlow
Therapy of Pain,
Lippincott, 1981

Edward Sylvester and Lynn C. Klotz
The Gene Age
Charles Scribner Sons, 1983

Drs. E. M. Todd, B. L. Crue, Jr., and M. Vergadamo
City of Hope Medical Center, California
Bulletin, Los Angeles Neurological Society
Vol. 30, No. 3, 1965

Dr. J. Unger
Technical University of Munich, Germany
CSF Somatostatin is Elevated in Patients with Postzoster Neuralgia
Neurology, September 1988

Drs. Abbas Vafai, Ronald S. Murray, Mary Wellish, Mary Devlin,
and Donald H. Gilden
University of Colorado School of Medicine
Expressions of Varicella Zoster Virus and Herpes Simplex Virus
in Normal Human Trigeminal Ganglia
Procedures of the National Academy of Sciences
Vol. 85, April 1988

Drs. Abbas Vafai, Mary Wellish and Donald H. Gelden
University of Colorado School of Medicine
Expression of Varicella Zoster Virus in Blood Mononuclear Cells
of Patients with PHN
Procedures of the National Academy of Science
Vol. 85, April 1988

Dr. Patrick D. Wall
Cerebral Functions Group
University College of London
Mechanism of Acute and Chronic Pain, 1984

Sir John Walton
Brains Diseases of the Nervous System
Oxford University Press, 1988

Dr. S. W. Wassilew
Dermatology Clinic
Krefeld, Republic of Germany
Oral Acyclovir for Herpes Zoster
British Journal of Dermatology
Vol. 117, 4, 1987

Dr. C. P. N. Watson
University of Toronto
Postherpetic Neuralgia Postmortem
Fifth World Congress on Pain,
Hamburg, Germany, August, 1987
Elsevier Science Publishers

Dr. Peter N. Watson
University of Toronto General Hospital
Postherpetic Neuralgia: A Review
Archives of Neurology, Vol. 43, 1986

Dr. Robert E. Weibel
Department of Virus and Cell Biology
Merck Sharp & Doehm
Live Attenuated Varicella Virus Vaccine
New England Journal of Medicine,
Vol. 310, 22, May 31, 1984

Dr. Richard J. Whitley
University of Alabama
Early Vidarbine Therapy to Control the Complications of
Herpes Zoster in Immunosuppressed Patients
New England Journal of Medicine, Vol. 307, No. 11, 1982

Harold Williams
Correspondence of Jonathon Swift
Oxford Clarendon Press, 1963

Dr. D. J. Winston
UCLA Medical Center

Recombinant Interferon for Treatment of Herpes Zoster
American Journal of Medicine, Vol. 85, No 2, 1988

Dr. M. S. Wood
East Birmingham Hospital, England
Efficacy of Oral Acyclovir Treatment of Herpes Zoster
American Journal of Medicine, Vol. 85, 2A, 1988

Dr. James B. Wyngaarden
Director, NIH,
Text book of Medicine
Harcourt Brace Jovanovitch, 1988